Managing Yourself

ESSENTIALS OF NURSING MANAGEMENT

Titles in the series

Annabel Broome: Managing Change, 2nd edition

Principles of complex change
Leadership and creating change from within
Imposed to change
The nurse as a change agent
Identifying training and development needs
Appendices

June Girvin: Leadership and Nursing

The development of theories of leadership
Interpretations of leadership
Interpersonal skills and leadership
Leadership and nursing
The story so far…
Traditional attitudes and socialisation
Motivation
Leadership today
Vision – foresight, insight and dreams

Diana Sale: Quality Assurance, 2nd edition

An introduction to quality assurance
Total quality management
Standards of care
Clinical audit
Clinical protocols
Monitoring of providers by purchasers

Verena Tschudin *with* **Jane Schober: Managing Yourself,** 2nd edition

'Know thyself'
Valuing yourself
Motivating yourself
Asserting yourself
Stressing yourself
Supporting yourself
Celebrating yourself
Developing yourself and your career

ESSENTIALS OF NURSING MANAGEMENT

Managing Yourself

2nd Edition

Verena Tschudin

with Jane Schober

MACMILLAN

First edition 1990
Reprinted three times
Second edition 1998
Published by
MACMILLAN PRESS LTD
Houndmills, Basingstoke, Hampshire RG21 6XS
and London
Companies and representatives
throughout the world

ISBN 0–333–73142–5

A catalogue record for this book is available
from the British Library.

This book is printed on paper suitable for recycling and made from fully managed and sustained forest sources.

10 9 8 7 6 5 4 3 2 1
07 06 05 04 03 02 01 00 99 98

Editing and origination by
Aardvark Editorial, Mendham, Suffolk

Printed in Malaysia

Contents

Acknowledgements

The author would like to thank Jane Schober very particularly for writing the last chapter again. Special thanks go to Richenda Milton-Thompson for her constant help and encouragement with this project.

Every effort has been made to trace all the copyright holders but if any have been inadvertently overlooked the publishers will be pleased to make the necessary arrangement at the first opportunity.

Preface

'Management' is one of those words that say very little and imply a great deal. As long as you manage, you're OK.

Management usually means 'other people'. In this book, it means yourself, and this is where the problem starts. We generally know how to manage others. We know what they should do, how they should behave, how they should do their job, look after their children, deal with their colleagues and so on. But to apply these same principles to ourselves is not nearly as easy.

This book starts with the principle that 'charity begins at home'. This does not mean indulging ourselves in all sorts of excess. It means, on the contrary, a kind of discipline that does not shrink away from looking at the good *and* bad in us, the strengths *and* weaknesses, the helpful *and* unhelpful, the possible *and* impossible parts of ourselves. This can sometimes be daunting. It is not easy to face up to the darker side of the reality that we are, or make choices that lead us into the unknown. However, it is often there that discoveries are made that can and will transform our lives.

As a nurse, you are first of all a *person*, and although addressed to you as a nurse, this book looks at you as a person. It is meant for you the person, to be more effective in your work as a nurse to manage yourself and others better.

VERENA TSCHUDIN
January 1998

Chapter 1 'Know thyself'

Awareness

'Know thyself' was written over the entrance to the temple of Apollo at Delphi. The oracle situated there normally gave obscure responses to requests. To 'know thyself' is a clear enough instruction but not simple to put into practice.

Nurses have a better idea of the intricate workings of the body than do most people, but nurses may not necessarily understand better than their patients and clients what the emotional, spiritual, social and psychological ramifications of illness and disease may be. Cancer, for example, is not just a disease; with it comes a whole package of emotions and questions about life and death, meaning, beliefs and existence.

Getting to know yourself is not necessarily painful. It *can* be painful, but essentially it is liberating.

Kevin

> Kevin was a lecturer in a college of nursing. This had led him to do a counselling course and had helped him to understand the power of symbols. One day, he said, 'I have gone through life like a snail: slow, cumbersome, and retreating often into my shell.' When a colleague pointed out that snails also leave a silvery trail behind them, this was like a revelation; he could see himself as having left something precious of himself. His life took on a more positive meaning.

Awareness and self-discovery are not ends in themselves. They are there to help you discover the wider meaning of life in general and your place in it in particular. They help you to get the maximum out of life.

We make an impact on life whether we like it or not. To know what that impact – that silvery line – is, we actually have to be

1

aware what kind of mark we make and where. We have to be aware – of the body, the emotions, the mind, the spirit, the environment. They shape us, but we shape them too.

All search for impact, for change and for success starts here and now. No book can give you interpersonal skills – you have them already – but this book aims to help you to become aware of, and to improve and utilise, your skills.

Awareness of the body

Most people criticise their bodies. Hair grows where it shouldn't, a muscle is too tight, a pain too limiting, the digestion too fast or too slow, the nails are not as attractive as someone else's. In order to use our bodies effectively, we need to co-operate with them rather than chastise them.

We influence our bodies with clothes, diet and exercise. We give our bodies an image with scents and ornaments, but our bodies are also influenced by biorhythms, by the time of day, the environment, our lifestyle and our character.

Wherever you are, stop now in the position in which you are. Notice the position of your body. Just notice it – don't change it.

- Are you comfortable? What is your position saying to you?
- What is your position saying about you to others?
- If you like, change your position to one more comfortable, significant, evocative.
- What would you most like to express at this moment with your body? Do it.

In order to learn more effective awareness of the body, try to:

- be aware without judging;
- acknowledge without criticising;
- accept without blaming.

When you are aware of your body, you are also aware of the space around it.

> The following took place at a tube station.
>
> A very pretty girl with noisy shoes went up to a smallish, middle-aged man wearing a cloth cap. In a loud voice she said, 'Hello, darling', then walked away. As a train pulled in, she made her way to the man again, going close up but saying nothing. Hastily, he walked to another carriage. The girl stood outside, laughing loudly at him.
>
> Do you know what your usual defence is when someone gets too close? Would you normally use words or body language to defend yourself? The interpretation that we give of our own and other people's behaviour shapes our lives much more significantly than we are aware most of the time.
>
> Awareness of the body is so basic that we tend to overlook its impact and take it for granted. The way we walk, talk and dress, what we eat and how, how we look at others and let them look at us: all these things say who we are, and we say to the world who and what we are – or what we think we are, or would like the world to think we are, or imagine that we are, or would like to be.

Awareness of the senses

The senses are the go-betweens between the outer world of the body and the inner world of the emotions, the mind, the psyche and the soul.

We often say 'I see', and this has nothing to do with the physical eyes and the sense of *seeing*, but with the 'inner eye', the perception.

When you meet a person you know in the street, you see that person, but with your inner eyes you 'see' past meetings with that person, and this colours your present behaviour. When you see a plate of pasta, you remember a time you had a plate of pasta: on a holiday in Italy, with a friend, or because you did not know what else to choose from the menu.

The physical senses are the parts of the person that locate you in the world, give meaning to your past and present, and shape your future. What happens in the outside world is interiorised by the senses in order to shape the personality.

3

The sense of *hearing* conveys a sound from the physical world to that of understanding and knowing. When you hear correctly, you can respond correctly, and it is in responding that we are 'humanised'. We express ourselves most truly when we respond to people, events and objects.

> Stop for a moment and become aware of all the sounds around you. Listen to them. Does any one sound mean anything in particular? If so, stay with that sound and its meaning for as long as feels appropriate.

'The way to a man's heart is through his stomach' is perhaps the best-known adage of the sense of *taste*. Whenever we celebrate something, we do so with food or drink. What do you eat or drink to celebrate? What interpretation do you give for this?

Some people who are very ill, especially patients who receive radiotherapy, lose their sense of taste. There is a correlation between losing the taste on the tongue and losing the taste for life.

> Think of your favourite food for a moment and be aware of the expression on your face, the flow of saliva and the flow of gastric juices this creates. Be aware of what you are saying to and about yourself with this.

The sense of *smell* is closely linked to taste. If you could never smell that the food you are cooking is in fact burning, you would not enjoy eating it either!

> Do you prefer the smell of tea or coffee? Don't give reasons, just stay with this simple choice as an exercise of awareness.

Touching, the last sense, is extremely important for nurses. There is a difference between giving an injection and giving an injection that will help the patient to get better.

A touch can be comforting and can also be hurtful. It can be given with meaning, as when holding someone close, or it can be constraining someone violent. A handshake will reveal cold, warm, sweaty or trembling hands and in this way give a good indication of that person's state of health or mind.

The sense of touch is something not only sensual, but also sensuous. The traditionally inhibited Britons are only too well aware of this. Touching, above all other senses, is surrounded by taboos. Touching someone with gloves on your hands gives protection but also creates distance. How, when and where do you touch a person who expresses a need to be touched?

Awareness of the environment

To be aware of the body means also to be aware of the environment. Without the earth's gravity, we would not be able to walk, and a person's first deed anywhere – in the kitchen, on the bus, in the ward – is to make an impact on that environment simply by walking into it.

The environment – the house you live in, the area you grew up in, the air you breathe, the newspaper you read, the way to work, the work you do, the places you go to for leisure – all these shape you and condition you to be the person you are. A patient who looks out on a park with a pond and flowers, who sees people picnicking and children playing, is likely to get better more quickly than one whose view is a brick wall without even any sky.

It has been said that you are what you eat, or read or wear. In the same way, you are what you look out on; you are what surrounds you, the places you visit, the house you live in. 'Your house is your larger body', writes Gibran (1926, p. 38).

Awareness of the environment may mean for one person the ability to have a garden, and for another the ability to be totally absorbed in a sunrise, to live in a high-rise flat, or to join the people protesting against another motorway. Nature and nurture have given us possibilities and values. In turn, we take those values and, by our lives, shape the environment for ourselves and others.

> Think for a moment:
>
> ● What aspect of the environment, near or far, makes a deep impression on you?
> ● What part of the environment have you yourself shaped?
> ● What part would you *like* to shape or change and how?

There are no right or wrong answers to such questions. What is right for you is the best, and only that matters. Simply taking note of something puts you in relation to it, and the relationship you have – the way you respond to her, him or it – makes you the person you are.

Awareness of temperament

In order to manage ourselves well, we need to know ourselves well. *Self-knowledge* develops as contacts with people develop. Differences become accentuated and preferences for acting in one way or another become clear.

There are many systems in use for defining people's temperaments and characteristics. Astrology is well known; Chinese horoscopes have become familiar in the West; and from olden times, people have been labelled according to the four body humours believed to exist – sanguine (blood), choleric (bile), melancholic (black bile) and phlegmatic (phlegm).

The psychologist C. G. Jung also found that people fall into four broad types: thinking, feeling, sensing and intuiting. These categories have been simplified and made accessible by Isabel Myers and her mother Katherine C. Briggs in what they call the Myers–Briggs Type Indicator. This will now be addressed in more detail and used throughout this chapter.

The Myers–Briggs Type Indicator

As you read through this outline of the Myers–Briggs Type Indicator (MBTI), try to see into which type you yourself fit most readily. The ideal would be that each of us would be capable of functioning equally well in all categories. The fact is that we have clear 'preferences' but with the equally clear possibility of developing the opposite, or **shadow**, quality.

Extraverted/introverted

The first distinction made in Myers–Briggs is the 'orientation' **extraversion (E)** or **introversion (I)**. The way to find out simply which you are is to ask yourself this question: do you get your energy from being with people or from being alone?

Extravert (E) people are sociable. They like to be with and around people, and they get very lonely when they are not surrounded. They are the life and soul of a party because they need (for their energy) to be the centre of attraction.

Elizabeth

> Elizabeth is 63 and was widowed about a year ago. She frequently turns up at the GP's surgery with different types of ailments and pains that never need much attention. She had been the youngest of six children, married early and worked with her husband in his design business at some distance from the rest of her family. They had no children but frequently joined in family gatherings. When her husband died of a heart attack, she found herself bereft of her life partner, driver and constant companion. Being alone for the first time in her life was almost worse than the loss itself.

Introvert (I) people, on the other hand, are very territorial. They need space around them, both physical space and mental space. They often pursue activities on their own as they recharge their batteries in this way. In a crowd, they can feel very lonely and disconnected, and after half an hour at a party they are ready to go home. They often work well *with* people, but it drains them.

No-one is totally either extraverted or introverted. Each needs the other, but the suppressed, or shadow, side is less obvious. In Western society, about 75 per cent of the population are extraverted (Keirsey and Bates, 1984, p. 25), which means that introverted people tend to have more difficulty in feeling accepted. To be told that it is 'OK' to be introverted can be a considerable relief for these people.

Sensing/intuitive

The main characteristics of the temperament are the 'functions': sensing and intuiting, thinking and feeling. Each person 'prefers' one of the functions in each pair.

To know, roughly, whether you are either a **sensing (S)** or **intuitive (N)** type – 'N' is used as 'I' already stands for introversion – ask yourself this: would you describe yourself mainly as a practical (S) or as an innovative (N) person? Do you prefer actualities (S) or possibilities (N)? It appears that sensing people constitute about 75 per cent of the population, and intuitives about 25 per cent (Keirsey and Bates, 1984, p. 25).

Sensing (S) people need things to be realistic. They trust experience, the past, down-to-earth facts and actuality. They are also very good at picking up details. In short, they trust anything that their senses have experienced. Small wonder, perhaps, that sensing people make good nurses, doctors and policemen.

Intuiting (N) people, on the other hand, are often described by others as having their heads in the clouds. They like what is possible, in the future. They will accept change as a challenge and are always interested in growth. While sensing persons see details, intuitives see wholes. They make connections, trust images and hunches, and enjoy metaphors and ideas. They are the inventors, innovators and pioneers, both in science and in the arts.

Briggs–Myers (1980, p. 58) believes that differences in national characteristics between the British and American can be described in terms of the differences between sensing and intuiting. The appeal of the New World drew the intuitives to the West like bees to honey, leaving a proportionally large share of sensing people in Britain to enjoy their afternoon tea, Beefeaters and long weekends!

Thinking/feeling

The next division is between **thinking (T)** and **feeling (F)**. Here, the division in the population is about half and half, although men tend to be the thinking, and women the feeling, types.

The simple question to ask yourself here is: do you prefer to make decisions based on personal impact (F) or on principle, logic or objectivity (T)?

Since the education system stresses all the aspects of thinking, people who are naturally feeling types often also have well-developed thinking capacities, whereas thinking types are less likely to have developed their feeling characteristics.

Thinking (T) people like words such as 'objectivity', 'principle', 'law', 'justice', 'analysis' and 'firmness'. To a *feeling* (F) person, words such as 'values', 'persuasion', 'personal', 'humane', 'harmony', 'appreciation' and 'devotion' are literally the stuff of life.

Feeling people will often label thinkers as cold, calculating, remote and heartless. Conversely, thinkers will label feeling people as emotional and illogical, and as wearing their hearts on their sleeves.

Both types of person experience feelings. The thinking types, however, tend not to show them but instead internalise them (which may perhaps account for the fact that more men than women have ulcers).

Because these functions are the only ones that are sex-related, the divisions of professions can be explained in terms of temperament: men tend to be employed as lawyers, managers, MPs and analysts, using their thinking function. Women, using their feeling function for social contact, predominate in work such as nursing, social work and counselling.

Judging/perceiving

The last pair is that of 'attitudes' to surroundings. Here, people are either **judging (J)** or **perceiving (P)**. (The words 'judging' and 'perceiving' can be misleading: 'judging' refers rather to concluding, 'perceiving' to 'becoming aware'.) In this case, the question to ask yourself to find out which type you are is this: do you prefer things to be closed and settled (J), or do you prefer to keep options open and fluid (P)? Do you always know which train you will catch (J), or do you go to the station and take whichever train happens to go (P)? There seems to be no clear distinction in the population for either of these types, and people are about evenly divided between them.

Judging (J) people like things settled, orderly, planned and completed. They plan ahead, make lists and follow them, and get things moving.

Perceiving (P) people, on the other hand, seem to 'play'. They do not like planning, preparing or clearing up. They are flexible, adapt as they go, are tentative and will delay making decisions, hoping always that something better will turn up.

Briggs–Myers (1980) describes the 'gifts' which each of these types has, the gifts of judgement being (among others) a system in doing things, order in possessions, sustained effort and acceptance of routine (p. 71). Some of the gifts of perception are spontaneity, open-mindedness, tolerance, curiosity and adaptability.

It may be difficult for you to decide into which of these two types you fall; with this pair in particular there is a sense of not knowing what is the natural tendency, what you should do and what you actually do. What you *naturally* do is the right choice.

Awareness of character traits

The conclusion from these simple outlines is that there is a great variety of both people and temperaments. Myers and Briggs have detailed 16 types. They are called by the letters corresponding to each of the significant words ESTP, ISTP, ENFJ, ISFP, ENTJ, INTP and so on.

The significance of this typing is in helping us to recognise a person's character traits. These determine his or her choices, values and way of living and acting. However, a simple outline of any system of categorising the temperaments cannot do justice to all the important elements of psychological typing. In particular, it cannot distinguish the significant aspects of personal, social and cultural background. The importance of the exercise is, however, to see the possibilities: you are the person you are because and in spite of all your personal luggage. Learning or knowing what is in the shadow for you gives you the power to develop your potentialities.

Amanda	

Amanda was an experienced F-grade nurse who got on well with her colleagues. However, she had difficulties with Sandra, one of the consultants. Amanda was, according to the Myers–Briggs Type Indicator, an ISFJ (introverted, sensing, feeling, judging). Her knowledge of the typing made her understand that Sandra was ESTP (extraverted, sensing, thinking, perceiving), almost the opposite of her.

I v. E: Amanda would often see herself as inferior to Sandra and would therefore not speak out when she really wanted to. Once she had not contradicted Sandra on a particular matter, she found it twice as hard to stand up to her the next time. Sandra, on the other hand, did not consider it necessary to ask whether Amanda had any questions: she assumed that everybody could speak their mind easily. This led to the first communication problems.

S: Both were sensing people, practical and observant of patients' conditions. At that level, they respected each other's work.

F v. T: Amanda would consider a patient's whole situation: seeing the person's illness, family, values expressed, the meaning given to the present predicament and the relationship that she and her staff had with the particular patient. Sandra would see a condition, a set of treatments and an outcome. She could not understand Amanda's ofen complicated descriptions. Amanda found Sandra cold and calculating.

One day, Amanda phoned Sandra to request that she come and visit a particular patient who was in great pain. Sandra promised to come within the hour. When four hours later she phoned to say she could not come until tomorrow, Amanda did not insist. She went home and tormented herself about her inability to make Sandra realise the urgency of the request.

J v. P: The judging function in Amanda made her value a job well finished, knowing that all was done before she started on something new or left work. Sandra, however, set no great store by deadlines, and when an unexpected situation turned up, she followed that. Sandra could never be pinned down, and this annoyed Amanda, although she recognised that that particular quality was valued by the patients with whom Sandra would sometimes spend a lot of time, never giving the impression that she had anything else to do.

Because Amanda knew her type, she was aware of her strengths, particularly her caring attitude with patients and staff. One of the characteristics was an even temper. She knew that some of this was due to her introversion. She found her biggest problem to be a strict judging attitude. This often led her to believe that others ought to be like her: tidy, methodical, always punctual and meaning what they said. However, she had to learn that not everybody was like that, and once she was able to see – with the help of an empathic friend – that she herself might gain by being less strict with herself, she found that she got on even better with other people, especially Sandra.

She was able to acknowledge Sandra's different characteristics as strengths and aimed to work with them rather than let herself be dominated by them. Sandra responded positively to this change by becoming less 'bossy' and more of a colleague.

An awareness of temperament can be a great help. The real help, however, is knowing what the *shadow*, the undeveloped part, is. Just as towards evening the sun casts longer shadows, so as we grow older our 'shadow' becomes longer and more apparent to ourselves and others. The challenge is to deal with it.

- If you have decided which type you are, what does that say to you?
- Now think of the person you live/work with most closely:
  – What type is that person according to this simple outline?
  – What are your main differences?

Look at them, and study the differences, particularly the positive sides. See what changes you might make to ease a tense situation.

Awareness of other people

'No man is an island' is another simple statement that takes a lifetime to unravel and come to grips with. Volumes have been written on who and what the 'other', the 'neighbour', is. We belong to each other and depend on each other. I would like to do no more here than simply raise the subject as a prelude to much allusion in this book to 'others'.

The objection to self-awareness put by many people is that it leads to introspection and self-centredness. This objection is mainly a fear and a distorted idea of self-awareness. True awareness leads not to selfishness but to a deeper understanding of people in general and of how relationships function. A true knowledge of self leads to a true knowledge of others.

One of the benefits of personality indicators is this knowledge of how other people function. To realise that another person has aims and needs, interests, feelings and values other than our own can and should release us from our own need to change the world and everything and everyone in it. Instead, we can get on with living the life we have more effectively and more content-edly – and *perhaps* help another to live his or her life more effectively too. We cease to be 'directors' of others and instead become 'enablers'.

Awareness of others will also lead to our being more at ease, knowing and accepting how others see us and how they respond to us and to our presentation of ourselves. In relation to awareness and self-knowledge, the answer to the question 'What's in it for me?' is 'A happier and more fulfilled life'. How this applies to your life depends on you and your interpretation of it. I hope that this book will help you to clarify what this *might* mean for you.

In order to manage yourself well, you need to be aware of yourself *and* all those things that surround you, your body *and* your feelings, your strengths *and* your shadowy needs. You have the choice to manage yourself or be managed (and used) by them, to be free yourself and to free others, or to be enslaved by yourself and all that surrounds you. To learn about this, the most important lesson is to become aware first without judging yourself. The practicalities of some of these issues are addressed in the pages that follow.

References

Briggs-Myers, I. (1980) *Gifts Differing*. Palo Alto, CA: Consulting Psychologists Press.

Gibran, K. (1926) *The Prophet*. London: Heinemann, 1980 edn.

Keirsey, D. and Bates, M. (1984) *Please Understand Me*. Del Mar, CA: Prometheus Nemesis.

Chapter 2 Valuing yourself

'You know what it is until someone asks you to define it', said St Augustine of time. The same can be said of much else in life. You think you know your values – until someone asks you what they are.

In this chapter and elsewhere in this book, I am outlining theories and viewpoints; some are other people's, but all are my own choice. I would like you to see them not as directives but as catalysts or pointers for your own choice of values and ideas.

Personal values

- Find a newspaper, magazine or journal that contains pictures.
- Without thinking and reflecting too much, quickly choose a picture that attracts you.
- What does the picture say about yourself?
- Does it evoke memories, depict how you feel, show you what you mean by (for example) beauty, invite you to imitate, give you a sense of peace?
- Settle on one reason why you have chosen this picture and revel in your choice.

Let the picture speak to you.

From the earlier outline of the temperaments, it can be seen that not everyone will find this exercise easy. Thinking people need facts, not imagination, to function. But all of us have **memories**, make **associations** and have **dreams** about the future. These three elements form the basis for the **esteem** in which we hold ourselves and the **values** we place on concepts and facts.

- What *memory* (for example of an illness or of your home life) has particularly shaped your life?
- What memory has particularly shaped a value that you hold?
- What *association* is now shaping your life? (Look again at your chosen picture. Does it evoke in you some current concern?)
- What association is shaping a value that you hold?
- What *dream* of the future is particularly shaping your life? (For example, you might wish to hold a certain job and are taking courses in the subject.)
- What dream of the future is particularly shaping a value for you?

Perhaps make a note of your answers and put the date by them. It may be interesting at a later date to see what has changed.

Viktor Frankl (1963) argues that the most important goal in life for a person is the search for **meaning**. He says that 'we can discover this meaning in life in three different ways: (1) by doing a deed, (2) by experiencing a value, (3) by suffering' (p. 113). Thus we have *creative* values, which we discover through doing or achieving; *experiential* values, which we discover by experiencing something such as a work of nature or culture – and also by experiencing someone; and *attitudinal* values, which we discover when confronted with something inescapable or unavoidable, such as our own and other people's suffering.

A point that Frankl makes strongly is that we *discover* the meaning of life and in life: we do not create it; hence the importance of awareness of ourselves, our surroundings and other people. Frankl illustrates this by saying that 'a cancer which can be cured by surgery must not be shouldered by the patient as though it were his cross. This would be masochism rather than heroism. But if a doctor can neither heal the disease nor bring relief to the patient by easing his pain, he should enlist the patient's capacity to fulfil the meaning of his suffering' (p. 115). This latter applies particularly also to nurses.

Values are changing elements in our lives. They are dynamic, and there is usually some motivation involved, but values are built on other factors, such as beliefs and attitudes.

Beliefs are often based on faith rather than facts. We believe that we are going to get home safely tonight; we have no facts to substantiate this.

Attitudes are settled dispositions. They are constant feelings that give order and shape to our lives. We have an attitude of caring, of gratitude, of courtesy. Such an attitude shows what kind of person someone is.

Values, then, are based on these two pillars. Because we believe that sick people should be cared for whatever their circumstances, we show this in the way we care. This care leads us to conform to certain rules, perhaps at some stage to challenge these rules because circumstances have changed and because we have changed through the care we have given. Our personal values (memories, associations and dreams) together shape our life: personal, societal and professional values cannot be separated. There may, however, be conflict when a *personal* value, such as protecting a colleague, who is also a friend but who may have harmed a patient, conflicts with a *professional* value, which demands that dangerous or harmful practice should be reported.

A person who values her or himself is a person of integrity, that is, someone who does not change with every wind of doctrine. This is certainly not easy in today's world. Part of managing yourself is therefore to have a value basis that you know and feel comfortable with.

- You might like to ask yourself, 'which basic values guide my life?' There may be more than one meaning, or you may not have a ready answer.
- You might like to stay with that question and your answer, as similar questions will come up throughout the book.

The values that you have noted on page 14 may also be applied to Frankl's creative, experiential and attitudinal values. You might like to consider your answers in the light of these categories.

Values that are right for one person are not necessarily right for another, hence the possibility of conflict. Values also emerge and change as we change and the world around us changes.

Social values. Many of our social values are formed because of fears. We are told that the environment will be destroyed if we use CFCs; our health will be affected if we eat beef (BSE), eggs (salmonella), chicken (antibiotic resistance) and sugar (dental caries). We are advised not to sit in the sun (skin cancer); not to go for a walk alone (fear of attack) and so on. Yet at every shop checkout, there are sweets and chocolates for last-minute buys, chicken is the cheapest protein, and the tourist industry promotes holidays in the sun.

Smith (1977, p. 69) lists eight questions that may help in clarifying how values come about:

1. Have I freely chosen this value?
2. From among what alternatives?
3. What are the consequences of choosing this value?
4. How recently have I acted on this value?
5. In what way has this value become a regular pattern in my life?
6. When did I most recently publicly affirm this value?
7. How do I prize or celebrate this value in my life?
8. How does this value help me to grow as a person?

The essence of these questions is that we have to *choose*, *prize* and *act* on values. We have to be aware of what is given, find the meaning of it and then do something about it.

What is here? What is happening?	} *Choosing*
What is the meaning of it? What is your purpose?	} *Prizing*
What are you doing about it?	*Acting*

Look at the following sentences and complete them, aware, as far as possible, of how you came to hold such a value, what its implications are and how you would defend it if asked:

- One day I hope to...
- My work is...
- People who are well dressed are...
- My favourite place is...
- Elderly people should...
- The person who influences me most taught me to...
- If I were ill I would...   *(cont'd)*

- Artistic beauty is...
- If I had a million pounds, I would...
- My parents are...
- Sick people are...
- I would like to be remembered for...
- The people I work with are...
- Developing and discovering means...
- My greatest possession is...
- I am lucky to have...
- Freedom of speech is...
- What I would most like to change is...

Having answered the questions, you might like to do this exercise again and see whether you would have answered these questions differently five years ago and what has changed for you in the meantime. You might also keep in mind that meaning is not created but discovered.

Professional values

Under this heading, I would like to highlight certain areas of nursing values that I find significant. Look at them critically, and check your own values against them.

Roach, who has written a great deal about caring, says in an early work (1984, p. 2) that 'caring is the locus of all attributes used to describe nursing'. **Caring** is thus not only the main *value* of nursing but its *essence*. However, she sees caring not only as a nursing act; she says that 'to care is human; to be human is to care'. She details her theory by establishing the 'Five Cs' of caring (Roach, 1992, p. 57):

- compassion
- competence
- confidence
- conscience
- commitment.

Compassion is 'a way of living born out of an awareness of one's relationship to all living creatures; engendering a response of participation in the experience of another; a sensitivity to the pain and brokenness of the other; a quality of presence which allows one to share with and make room for the other' (p. 58).

Competence is 'the state of having the knowledge, judgement, skills, energy, experience and motivation required to respond adequately to the demands of one's professional responsibilities' (p. 61).

Confidence is 'the quality which fosters trusting relationships' (p. 62).

Conscience is 'a state of moral awareness; a compass directing one's behaviour according to the moral fitness of things' (p. 63).

Commitment is 'a complex affective response characterised by a convergence between one's desires and one's obligations, and by a deliberate choice to act in accordance with them' (p. 65).

Campbell (1984) adds another dimension to nursing, which, coincidentally, also begins with C: he describes nursing as **companionship**:

The good companion is someone who shares freely but does not impose, allowing others to make their own journey... Companionship is bodily presence, but not specifically sexual... The good companion looks ahead and encourages... The commitment of companionship is a *limited* one... parting is an essential element in companionship. (pp. 49–50)

If nursing can be summed up as 'caring', and caring is the human mode of being, nurses should above all be human: 'An individual cares, not because he or she is a nurse, but because he or she is a human being' (Roach, 1984, p. 2). Caring in nursing is unique precisely because nursing is above all a profession in which being human is so important:

In the current economic climate and competitive market place of health care, the nursing profession must promote the caring aspects of their role to distinguish themselves from others and secure a future as major contributors to high quality patient care. Caring for and about patients must be valued and be made a more visible part of what nurses have to offer. (McKenna, 1993)

- How do you respond to these statements?
- Do they represent the values you have of nursing, of yourself as a nurse and as a person?
- What would you change or add? Make a note of it.

In order to translate these theories into practice, I would like to examine briefly just four areas of nursing that are particularly relevant today.

Professionalism

'The concepts of profession, professionalism and professionalization are surrounded to some extent by conflicting views and controversy' (Jolley, 1989, p. 8). These concepts are, like many other such values, changing and adapting, and need constantly to be redefined in the light of new issues. Professionalisation used to be seen as something positive, with a clear knowledge base, and well organised internally. Davies (1996a) sees this as a male-oriented cloak to maintain the 'mastery' of relevant knowledge and being in command. This is not relevant to nursing practice. She suggests that there is 'another approach to knowledge, one that sees it as confirmed in use, that values things other than the formal and abstract, copes with uncertainty, acknowledges the intuitive and accepts the importance of experience' (Davies, 1996b).

It would be difficult to put these things into a code. Yet all practising nurses, midwives and health visitors are required to observe the UKCC *Code of Professional Conduct* (1992). In daily practice, nurses also have to consider a great number of policies and principles of good practice. In an effort to clarify some of these, the UKCC has published *Guidelines for Professional Practice* (1996). This states that 'the code sets out:

- the value of registered practitioners;
- your responsibilities to represent and protect the interests of patients and clients; and
- what is expected of you.

A code is not a piece of legislation; it cannot protect a person, and it cannot be a guide in specific situations. Each nurse, midwife and health visitor has to interpret the Code individually in given circumstances.

> - How well do you know the UKCC Code?
> - When and how do you use the Code?
> - Has it shaped your professional values?
> - Do you think your patients and clients should know of the Code?
> - How would it enable them to know the Code?

May (1975) develops another dimension of professionalism: the idea of **covenant.** According to him, a covenant is 'an original experience of gift between... partners'. Code and covenant are similar materially, but they differ in spirit. Contracts and codes define relationships, but covenants 'have a gratuitous growing edge to them that nourishes rather than limits relationships'... Contracts are external; covenants are internal to the parties involved.' In contracts, there is a tit-for-tat; in covenants, one *gives*. This is what Roach (1984) is pointing to when she says that to care is human. To be human one has to be creative; giving – responding – is creative.

> In the light of these theories, you might like to formulate your own list of professional values.
>
> As an example:
> - When I am caring, I...
> - As a nurse, I...
> - As myself, I...

Maybe you would like to say that when you are really caring for someone you are most fulfilled, but are these the words you use when you tell your friends about your work? Are there differences in what you would answer to these questions when you are alone and when you are with others? If so, what might be the reasons, and what might be the differences?

Advocacy

Curtin (1979) bases a philosophy of nursing on the concept of **advocacy**. She says that an advocate is first and foremost a person who can and does enter into a relationship with another person. Caring relationships are based on human rights, and these in turn derive from human needs. The human rights of life and liberty, and the pursuit of justice, happiness, truth, knowledge, beauty, harmony and so on, are needs. Too often, however, needs are confused with wants.

Advocacy implies interest and partnership. When nurses act as advocates, they claim to act in the patient's best interests. Precisely what the patient's best interests are is not always very clear. The phrase 'Good health is in John's interest and John has an interest in good health' has often been used to distinguish between the two uses of the word 'interest'. Most situations are not totally clear cut, so 'it is not possible, nor morally required, to respect every desire that people have, especially since some desires may be evil' (Ellis, 1996). To be truly an advocate, one would have to be independent of the system. This is not possible for nurses. In most nursing situations, advocacy does not mean *representing* a person but with every means possible helping that person to be not dependent (and perhaps frightened) but informed and 'self-advocating'.

'Advocacy also involves providing support if the patient refuses treatment/care or withdraws consent' (UKCC, 1996, p. 13). This may mean that nurses respect a decision even when they cannot agree with it. However, advocacy means perhaps more often defending patients against unwanted treatments and perhaps standing up to bully-tactics and rudeness (Mort, 1996) or ignorance (Kohner, 1996) from colleagues. When people are ill and perhaps handicapped, they are vulnerable in several different ways. To be taken advantage of or be disrespected should not be added. The advocate therefore becomes the partner of vulnerable, defenceless and perhaps endangered people. This can give nurses a sense of power, but also a sense of identity, which may not always be very healthy. The motives for acting in the patient's best interests must therefore be clearly thought through.

Pam

After her lumpectomy, Pam was told that she would need chemotherapy. But she felt very strongly that she did not want this. She discussed with her nurse what she should do to get across to the consultant that she did not want chemotherapy. The nurse stayed with her while she told the doctor of her decision and confirmed that they had talked about this in detail beforehand.

(Tschudin, 1994, pp. 82–4)

- Should the nurse have acted as he did?
- What do you think you would have done in this case?
- Have you had some similar experience?
- What did you mainly gain/learn/suffer from such an experience?

Advocacy is not a new concept or slogan; it is one of the basic values of nursing. However, the conflicts that it may bring are not easy to resolve. The issues of personal responsibility and awareness of values and meaning are sharply focused here. New concepts, such as self-advocacy (primarily used by minority or underprivileged groups to get a voice) and citizen advocacy (ordinary people being involved with vulnerable individuals) may also need to be studied and learnt. Perhaps the most important element in advocacy is listening and really hearing what the patient or client is actually saying.

- Where in your work is advocacy used, or questioned or abused?
- How much priority do you give to advocacy?
- Do you see nursing values as, generally, growing or eroding?
- What are you doing to maintain and foster any particular values?

Accountability

'In the exercise of your professional accountability [you] must...' (UKCC, 1992). The word accountability has crept into the language, linked to professsionalism, and it is not clear exactly what is meant by it. If it simply means one more line of hierarchy, it is clearly not addressing the spirit of accountability. Hunt (1991) suggests that when a new idea or key word appears, it is useful to ask 'Who is promoting it and why? What is it about the economic/political/moral environment that makes this idea necessary or plausible now? What exactly does it mean? What does it mean for me, for my work, and the people I serve through my work?'

Fromer (1990) says that 'professional accountability can be divided into four more or less equal components: self, client, employing institution and society'. Marks-Maran (1993) lists four different areas of accountability: legal, managerial, professional and moral; in reverse order, these correspond to the former components. It is clear, however, that these different parts overlap. Without a basic moral accountability (demanding a self-awareness), there could not be adequate accountability in other areas of work. Accountability is the outcome of responsibility, and responsibility is the use of the ability to respond to others, notably clients and patients. May (1975) states that 'covenant fidelity to the patient remains unrealized if it does not include proficiency'.

This relates to the 'Five Cs' of caring (compassion, competence, confidence, conscience and commitment) and means, in effect, that one is able to give an account for having acted in a certain way. It brings us back also to self-awareness, to knowledge, to one's values of the meaning of nursing and to our own understanding and goal of life, of care, of suffering and of where our personal responsibility lies.

- What value do you place on accountability?
- Where in your caring are you particularly accountable?
- How does this manifest itself?
- Are you satisfied with this?
- If not, what might you or should you do to change it?

Whistleblowing

Whistleblowing has increasingly become an issue in nursing because of the widening gap between practitioners and managers. The UKCC *Code of Professional Conduct* (1992) specifies in several clauses that nurses 'must report to an appropriate person or authority' any actions or omissions which jeopardise patient and practitioner safety. The *Guidelines for Professional Practice* (1996) are even more specific (pp. 21–2), acknowledging that nurses may be 'afraid to speak out for fear of losing your job', which was the lot of several nurses who had blown the whistle.

The biggest problem with whistleblowing is a possible breach of confidentiality. For nurses, the other problem is that they are bound by the *Code of Professional Conduct* (1992), whereas a manager, to whom a matter may be reported, may not be bound in the same way (if he or she is not a nurse). The 'appropriate person or authority' may not be so 'appropriate' in given circumstances.

Whistleblowing is linked closely to advocacy, but this raises the issue of *loyalty*. Is a nurse first of all loyal to the patient (for whom she or he cares), to the doctor (who prescribes treatments), to the hospital or institution (which employs her or him) or to the profession (which controls her or his registration)?

The issue is largely surrounded by negatives: be careful, keep your head down, you may lose your job, you may be dismissed and so on. Apparently, only one NHS Trust has a 'Whistle-blower's Charter' (Waters, 1995). The fact that pressure groups like 'Public Concern at Work' and 'Freedom to Care' have increasing workloads perhaps speaks for itself.

In the name of accountability and advocacy, nurses will come into conflict with various aspects of their work. The duty of care demands also a duty to be 'politically responsive' (Albarran, 1995). This requires courage. It means also that nurses have to be confident in their practice, use skills of negotiation and canvassing, and understand how power is used as a means to influence change.

- What issues would cause you to blow the whistle?
- If you have blown the whistle, what is your main memory of the act?
- If you had to help a colleague in similar circumstances, what advice would you give her or him?
- What have you learned in particular from your experience?

There are many other professional issues that are value laden. Confidentiality, informed consent, private health care and complementary medicine are only some aspects that would need much attention. In your own area of work there will be other issues with their own values.

This chapter may have highlighted certain concerns for you that need further attention. The following chapters consider various aspects of dealing with personal and professional issues that nurses everywhere face from time to time.

References

Albarran, J.W. (1995) 'Should nurses be politically aware?' *British Journal of Nursing* 4(8): 461–5.

Campbell, A.V. (1984) *Moderated Love*. London: SPCK.

Curtin, L.L. (1979) 'The nurse as advocate: a philosophical foundation for nursing.' *Advances in Nursing Science* 1(3): 1–10.

Davies, C. (1996a) 'Cloaked in a tattered illusion.' *Nursing Times* 92(45): 44–6.

Davies, C. (1996b) 'A new vision of professionalism.' *Nursing Times* 92(46): 54–6.

Ellis, P. (1996) 'Exploring the concept of acting "in the patient's best interests".' *British Journal of Nursing* 5(17): 1072–4.

Frankl, V. (1963) *Man's Search for Meaning*. London: Hodder & Stoughton.

Fromer, M. (1990) 'Ethical issues in nursing care' in Tingle, J. 'Accountability and the law: how it affects the nurse'. *Senior Nurse* 10(2): 8–9.

Hunt, G. (1991) 'Professional accountability.' *Nursing Standard* 6(4): 49–50.

Jolley, M. (1989) 'The professionalization of nursing: the uncertain path' in Jolley, M. and Allan, P. (eds) (1989) *Current Issues in Nursing*. London: Chapman & Hall, pp. 1–21.

Kohner, N. (1996) *The Moral Maze of Practice; A Stimulus for Reflection and Practice*. London: King's Fund.

McKenna, G. (1993) 'Caring as the essence of nursing practice.' *British Journal of Nursing* **2**(1): 72–4.

Marks-Maran, D. (1993) 'Accountability', in Tschudin, V. (ed.) *Ethics: Nurses and Patients*. London: Scutari, pp. 121–34.

May, W.F. (1975) 'Code, covenant, contract, or philanthropy.' *Hastings Center Report* **5**: 29–38.

Mort, L. (1996) 'Critical of care.' *Nursing Times* **92**(19): 40–1.

Roach, M.S. (1984) *Caring: the Human Mode of Being, Implications for Nursing*. Perspectives in Caring Monograph 1. Toronto: University of Toronto.

Roach, M.S. (1992) *The Human Act of Caring; A Blueprint for the Health Professions*, 2nd edn. Ottawa: Canadian Hospital Association Press.

Smith, M. (1977) *A Practical Guide to Value Clarification*. La Jolla, CA: University Associates.

Tschudin, V. (1994) *Deciding Ethically; A Practical Approach to Nursing Challenges*. London: Baillière Tindall.

UKCC (1992) *Code of Professional Conduct for the Nurse, Midwife and Health Visitor*, 3rd edn. London: UKCC.

UKCC (1996) *Guidelines for Professional Practice*. London: UKCC.

Waters, J. (1995) 'Whistle while you work.' *Nursing Times* **91**(38): 18.

Chapter 3 Motivating yourself

Your values will eventually manifest themselves – your **motives** may not. They remain your private property. This is why they are so elusive yet so crucial: your management of yourself depends on them. The following story tries to elucidate where motivation comes from.

> A man was walking along a river when he saw a person coming towards him in the river, about to drown. The man pulled the person out and resuscitated him. As he walked on, another victim, about to drown, was in the river, and he helped this one out too. And so on with a third and fourth. After this he got up, to the astonishment of the onlookers, who chided him for not rescuing all the victims who were coming downstream. As he walked away, the man said, 'I am going upstream to see who or what throws the people in.'
>
> (Egan and Cowan, 1979, p. 140)

Motivation

What makes you get up in the morning and not sleep on? Is it the call of duty or hunger, or a meeting you are looking forward to? The alarm clock waking you up is the external stimulus; the internal stimulus is some drive, some hope, some call, some need.

Motivation has been described as 'the tendency of the organism to reduce its needs or to return to its state of equilibrium' (Stones, 1966, p. 97). This is too mechanistic a view. We do not eat only in order to quench hunger. We eat also for desire, for circumstances and for feelings.

O'Connor (1968, p. 31) lists some of the general reasons for motivation:

- genuine interest
- a wish to perform the task well
- conforming to a standard
- looking for approval from superiors
- looking for recognition from colleagues
- in order to please
- in order not to disappoint
- a better salary if success is achieved.

How often have we heard patients say something like, 'I can't die until my son graduates', 'They still need me at work' or 'I won't die until I've solved the problem with my daughter.' The common thread running through these statements is the belief that people can exert some influence over the course of their disease and life.

Motivation consists of both external and internal factors. An external weighing up of a situation, making an **estimate**, leads to an internal situation of **esteem**. That in turn leads to the response that characterises a person.

van Hooft (1995) speaks of traits and instincts in the formation of character. However, he says:

before we go on to ask whether our own internal states and motivations might be explained by our genes, we should note that there is a subtle shift in categories as we move from talk of instincts and traits to talk of dispositions, inclinations, motivations, and finally, desires. This shift corresponds to an increase in the possibility of reflexivity and self-consciousness. (p. 52)

The stimulus for the man who resuscitated people was presumably that he was fed up with resuscitating people. This led him to question what he was doing. His esteem for himself and the drowning people made him get up and do something positive. Knowing how slowly and laboriously institutions move, it may then have taken him a long time to achieve his goal that no more people were thrown in, but this will not have deterred him. His goal was worth the effort.

29

From the estimate to the esteem, from an external stimulus to the carrying out of an action, may be a long road. The self-respect that is generated is based in that feeling of being of value, and out of that comes the response to the stimulus.

- What are motivators for you? (Examples include a certificate, a gift and the knowledge of having done right.)
- When were you last motivated to make a significant break or change? What was the stimulus? Did it see you through the change?

Lucy

Lucy was a shy 16-year-old who was underweight and often sick. A well-meaning neighbour gave her a leaflet about pilgrimages to Lourdes, and Lucy's parents – in an effort to try everything – paid for her to go. There she mingled with sick people of all ages, some very handicapped. They all, however, looked well. Lucy became more companionable, decided to train as a nurse, and years later still used her memory of the looks on the pilgrims' faces to give herself and her patients courage.

- What was your reason or motive for going into nursing?
- What keeps you there now? (You might like to make a note of it.)
- What or which personal or professional value do you recognise as motivating you most in your work as a nurse?
  - money/security;
  - the need to be needed;
  - an impossibility of changing jobs;
  - exerting control;
  - influencing others;
  - giving of yourself to others;
  - being looked up to;
  - altruism; following the example of a charismatic person.
- Can you identify a particular standard that you want to or have to maintain?
  - a standard of care;
  - self-respect;
  - respect for others;
  - control;
  - justice;
  - autonomy;
  - honesty.

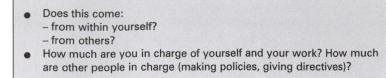

- Does this come:
  - from within yourself?
  - from others?
- How much are you in charge of yourself and your work? How much are other people in charge (making policies, giving directives)?

The man in the story at the start of this chapter changed from responding to what was simply there, to responding to a deeper insight. That must have changed the whole direction of his life. Once he had gone upstream he had some control over what he was doing – before then the situation had controlled him.

You may have known your values and acted on them. If and when you are confronted with a choice at some stage, you may simply not recognise your value or know your 'mind'. Your motives may be unclear. Your meaning, your 'leitmotiv', is questioned. This may be more of a challenge than a disaster. Like the rescuer, you may suddenly discover what lies potentially within you.

Mistakes and failures

Mistakes may be painful for all concerned. With every good intention, we still make mistakes, and skilled as we are at certain tasks, we still fail. Mistakes and failures then become positive or negative motivators. We either change or drift into apathy.

D. H. Lawrence is supposed to have said this: 'If only one could have two lives: the first in which to make one's mistakes, which seem as if they have to be made; and the second in which to profit by them.' We often learn more from our mistakes than in any other way. The learning comes when it is interiorised, acknowledged and owned.

- What big mistake(s) have you made in your life?
- If you look back to the temperament that you recognise, can you see the mistake(s) in terms of the undeveloped part of yourself (the shadow)?

(cont'd)

- What has been the main learning you have gained from a particular mistake?
- If you feel you have *not* learned from the mistake(s), what might you do now to turn it or them into a gain?
- Is there any mistake that you make often?
- Do you recognise any pattern or trait that leads up to making that mistake?
- Do you see a motivation for making the mistake? Do you see a motivation for changing your behaviour and avoiding the mistake? You might need to have support and help (see Chapter 6) with this.

The basis of mistakes and failures

The temperament (in the terms of the Myers–Briggs Type Indicator) is an important element in the understanding of mistakes and failures.

Sensing (S) people put much emphasis on history, past events and facts. They tend to dwell on their past and can recount and relive events leading up to an accident or disaster over and over again. Their intuitive personality is in the shadow, and therefore they do not trust the future and will rather stay with 'the devil they know'.

Intuitive (I) people on the other hand have a poor memory for history, and they will get up and go forward. Consequently, they may be inclined not to learn from mistakes because they pay little attention to the past.

Our personalities are shaped by our association with other people and with the environment in which we live and work. We are influenced and we let ourselves be influenced. We know this and realise it, but often we do not acknowledge it.

When we make **mistakes**, we make them out of the shadow, out of that part of the personality that is not well developed, known or controlled. This is why we get so furious when we make a mistake: we recognise that the mistake shows up the infantile, weak, incompetent and undeveloped part of ourselves.

Failure is different. A mistake has to be admitted; failure has to be lived with. Neither mistakes nor failures are wrong, or wrong-doing. However, a deliberately wrong action cannot be called a mistake: it is more than that.

A failure is, on the whole, not based on a particular mistake but rather on a series of events that have negatively influenced a person. The people in the story who were about to drown could be described as failures: failures of their own values and hopes, failures of the system in which they found themselves. Yet people in themselves are not failures; that would be to condemn them. However, events around them have influenced their behaviour and particularly their will – their motivation – and, rather than struggle forward, they have taken the easy way and drifted down with the tide.

- Where in your life have you had a failure?
- Can you remember what it felt like then?
- What, if anything, helped you to live with it?
- Do you describe something as a failure which others may not call that?
- How do you deal with other people who have made mistakes or have failed?
- Do you use different standards for you and for them?
- What do you think might be the reason for that?
- What one thing would you like to change in your life with regard to failures and mistakes?
- What stops you from doing so?

Judging a failure as such – in ourselves and others – is subjective. The values we place on making judgements, on failures and on successes, will colour any outcome.

We have to live with past failures, but we do not have to live and *perpetuate* a failure. Failures need to be seen in perspective, as a natural part of human living and growing. Like mistakes, they can be incentives to change, adapt and learn. Because they have to do with the shadowy, undeveloped part of ourselves, failures give us a possibility either of developing that side of ourselves or of further strengthening the strong part of the personality. Either possibility can be right at the right time.

- Do you think your failures have helped you in any way?
- Can that help which you received be used to help others?
- One metaphor used for this experience is that of 'the wounded healer'. Are you, or have you ever been, a wounded healer?

Renewed motivation

Mistakes and failures are painful. They lead to dark times in life when we feel dejected, lonely and helpless. They lead to loss of confidence and make us question any motives we had.

Yet such times also seem essential. When values become uncertain, when skills are doubted and when any self-esteem is absent, that is the moment when we are faced with ourselves. The question 'What is the meaning of it?' is then the only relevant question. As light has meaning only in darkness, so the real meaning of life is usually discovered only in a crisis. Once the meaning of something is discovered, the motivation for change, for direction or for defying any predictions is there. But change does not happen on its own. We have to take a personal responsibility for it.

To look only on the painful side of life is not enough. Ideally, the next step should now be some celebration of your achievements. This will be considered in Chapter 7. If you would like to work on this chapter next, be aware of your choice and your reasons for doing so or not doing so.

References

Egan, G. and Cowan, R.M. (1979) *People and Systems*. Belmont, CA: Brooks/Cole.

O'Connor, K. (1968) *Learning: An Introduction*. London: Macmillan, p. 31.

Stones, E. (1966) *An Introduction to Educational Psychology*. London: Methuen.

van Hooft, S. (1995) *Caring; An Essay in the Philosophy of Ethics*. Niwot, CO: University Press of Colorado.

Chapter 4 Asserting yourself

An assertive person is one who gets his or her needs and wants met without stepping on the rights of others. (Egan, 1977, p. 267)

Tact is a method of putting your foot down without treading on anyone's toes. (Anon)

Assertiveness has come to the fore with the feminist movement and is sometimes seen to be something peculiar to women. In practice, however, this is not true. Many men do not know how to use assertiveness, being more familiar with a commanding and aggressive type of behaviour.

Being assertive is nothing more and nothing less than being a good communicator. It is using oneself and the other person in such a way that both are enhanced and valued. When this happens, good management of human resources has taken place.

Aggression or assertion?

Assertiveness has to do with expressing feelings, needs, wants and rights. Egan (1977, p. 78) says that there are three different ways in which people express their emotions:

1. non-assertively – you just take it;
2. aggressively – you teach him a lesson;
3. assertively – you let him know how you feel without punishing him.

Bond (1986, p. 100) lists four approaches to expressing yourself:

1. assertive;
2. aggressive;

3. manipulative;
4. submissive;

These stances can also be expressed in transactional analysis (TA) language (Harris, 1973):

- I'm not OK – you're OK (submissive).
- I'm not OK – you're not OK (aggressive).
- I'm OK – you're not OK (manipulative).
- I'm OK – you're OK (assertive).

Each of these approaches is legitimate in its right setting. A person does not always need to get her or his way, have the last word or make others submit. Courtesy and manners, sometimes a dose of humility (not humiliation), and letting things be as they are, are also called for. However, when none of these approaches is constructive, assertiveness usually is.

The **submissive** way of being is one of appeasing. 'Would you mind…?', 'I mean, could you possibly…?', 'If I asked you nicely…?', 'Forgive me…': this is flattering the other, making her or him big and yourself small. We imagine that a 'big bully' will respond to us better if we enhance this bigness.

Being **passive** is taking things lying down, giving in. Even though we feel strong emotions, we say nothing. Later, however, we may burst into tears and in this way ensure that we are noticed and can tell our hard-luck story, blaming everyone and everything.

The **indirect** or **manipulative** approach can be hurtful but does not wound. It is an underhand, backlashing way, revealing an insecure personality. Double messages may be given: too friendly, too secure, too concerned. However, when it is all over, what remains is guilt – in the other person of course. People never quite know how to approach such a person, because he or she never 'comes clean' in any situation.

The **aggressive** person bloats herself or himself up to twice the size, hands on hips. The body language alone would say everything, but that is not enough: shouting, long tirades and verbal abuse are also the stock-in-trade to get what is wanted. Those around are careful (submissive) in case they provoke such a person even further. This alienates everybody, making each think that they are right and everybody else is wrong.

The **assertive** way of being and responding to emotions is everything else. You know what is going on, you remain cool, people do what you ask because you respect them – and they respect you. You do not *blame* others for what happens to you. You know what you need and want. If you are refused something, you are not demolished by it. You can respond to criticism because you can judge how valid it is.

Harris (1973) says that these stances are developed very early in life. The baby needs its mother: the baby is not OK but the mother who feeds and changes it is OK. There comes a time when the baby needs the mother but she lets the baby cry and does not pick it up: the baby is not OK, needing help, but the mother denies this – she is not OK either. The child learns to walk and be independent: the child becomes OK, but the parent constantly tells it not to do this or that he or she cannot have that – the parent is definitely not OK. Very much later in life – perhaps only in middle age – a person learns to be OK from deep within and to accept that other people are also OK. We thus grow up with behaviours and images learned and acquired in very black-and-white situations. The problems appear because, in life, most situations are more grey and intricate, but our patterns have not changed, at least not sufficiently. Most people and situations are, however, not as simple as this outline, but it may help to shed light on some behaviour and some relationships.

- Do you recognise yourself in any one of these roles? They may all apply at different times.
- Do you recognise in yourself a pattern for acting in one way more than another?
- Do you recognise any motives (see Chapter 3) for repeating any mistakes? Be aware of them and acknowledge them. You can only change what you know; when you know something, you have a lever for action.

In order to clarify any unproductive types of behaviour, it is useful to look at feelings, body language, needs, rights and wants in turn. In this way, you may see where you may want or need to make adjustments in your own style of communication.

Aspects of behaviour

Feelings

Feelings are powerful – and delicate – things, which can either make or mar a relationship. Feelings are experienced in the body but expressed in words – or not, as the case may be.

Letting feelings rule you altogether means that you are either in the clouds, down in the dumps or verbally abusive. Neither approach by itself is ideal; but as usual, a middle way would be preferable.

One simple method of finding this middle way is to learn how to distinguish feelings, how to express them and what other words we might find for similar feelings. Table 4.1 may help you with this. Please add to the lists your own appropriate words.

Table 4.1 Different types of feelings and different strengths of expression of feelings

	Happy	Sad	Angry	Confused
Strong	excited	hopeless	furious	bewildered
	elated	depressed	seething	troubled
Moderate	cheerful	upset	annoyed	disorganised
	merry	distressed	mad	mixed up
Weak	glad	sorry	uptight	bothered
	pleased	bad	irritated	undecided

(adapted from Tschudin, 1989, p. 48)

When you can *name* a thing – a feeling – you have some control over it. This does not mean suppressing it: feelings of deep sorrow are best expressed through tears, feelings of deep joy through laughter.

Feelings are simply there. They cannot be explained, and they cannot be explained away. A typical mistake is to counter them with reason.

Anna

> Anna, a GP practice nurse (and a feeling-type person), saw the need for some small changes to the appointments system they had recently introduced. She suggested that, in this way, everybody, patients, nurses, doctors and receptionists alike, would benefit. Jon, the senior partner (a thinking-type person), listened to her but did not believe that the changes would make any difference. Anna tried again, but as Jon shook his head, she sighed, 'If only you would be a bit more feeling!' This annoyed him, and he walked off with, 'If only you would learn to be logical!'

- Are you aware of any feelings that you often meet in yourself?
- Are your feelings shared by others?
- What do you do with your feelings when you are aware of them?

Once you are aware of your feelings, you can choose what to do with them: express them or control them. That choice is the most important element. Assertiveness in particular, and communication skills in general, are based on the ability to make that choice.

The further choice is between *sharing* your emotions and *releasing* them.

> Your colleague says to you, 'You've filled that form in wrong again. Can't you ever get anything right?'
>
> Your choice in answering is between:
>
> 1. 'I feel hurt and put down. I spent a lot of time filling in this form.'
> 2. 'Don't you shout at me! You don't know what you do to people with these remarks of yours.'

The release of emotion can happen in a controlled or uncontrolled way. You know what you are doing and saying, or you are flying off the handle. Anger in particular is often expressed in an uncontrolled way but then lasts only a short while before it is burnt up. Swallowed, however, it may go on for many years, poisoning the person and her or his environment.

- Which is your most usual way of dealing with strong emotion?
- Are you content with this, or would you like to change?
- What changes might you need to make?
- Make a note of the changes you might like to make, and in the light of this chapter see how you might bring this change about.

Body language

Assertiveness is about communication. **Body language** is the most basic and most obvious way we have of communicating.

Be aware right now of how you are sitting or standing. What is this posture saying to you and about you?

If possible, look at someone near you and notice what their body language is saying to you.

Our gestures often speak louder about us and for us than do our words. Our bodies reveal our thoughts, our attitudes and our desires. We can let them do this consciously, but in moments of crisis, they do it without our knowing. Here are some common expressions of feelings:

- In embarrassment, people may cover their mouths.
- In anger, they may lean forward.
- In sadness, they may turn sideways.
- When encroached upon, they may move back.
- When thinking hard, they may put their tongues out a little.
- When experiencing envy, they may become 'green'.
- When being submissive, they may bend at the knee.
- When talking deeply, they may look away.

Feelings may be swallowed or 'hidden', but the body can reveal them more than words can. People who are anxious or embarrassed often giggle. People put on an air of relaxation when they are seething with rage. To give such confused or mixed messages can be deliberate or unconscious.

> ● Do you make a particular gesture often?
> ● What do you think is a non-assertive way of standing?
> ● Take on that pose and feel what it is like. Do you recognise it as being familiar to you?

Patients are people under stress. They may therefore not behave 'as themselves'. As the person caring for them, you do not know what patients were like before they became ill; you have only the present to go by. How good are you at interpreting their put-on signals, their masks or their defences?

As a nurse, you are a privileged person: few family members can or would *touch* a person all over the body. You have the patient's unspoken (usually) agreement to invade her or his space. Some people welcome this; others resent it. The personal and cultural messages given with touch are particularly important in this area of body language.

> When you are caring for a patient, are you aware of the signals you are giving with your face when there is odour, disfigurement, like or dislike? Patients enjoy nothing so much as 'nurse-watching'.

Needs

Needs are another knowledge base for effective assertion. Consider the following text:

In Africa, they say that there are two hungers, the lesser hunger and the greater hunger. The lesser hunger is for the things that sustain life, the goods and services, and the money to pay for them, which we all need. The greater hunger is for an answer to the question 'why?', for some understanding of what that life is for. (Handy, 1997, p. 13)

Some needs are basic to life, constituting our lesser hunger. Generally we think that we can only have the higher hunger when all lesser hunger is satisfied. This may not necessarily be the case. People in hospital in particular, or those who are disabled or handicapped, may be acutely aware of both hungers. It may be difficult for nurses to know to which hunger they should respond.

Our needs constantly change.

Consider which hunger you are aware of. What is your need at this moment:

● to make a cup of coffee?
● to get the electrician to fix the faulty plug?
● to phone a friend and tell her or him what sort of a day you had?
● to finish reading this book?
● to compose the poem that has been growing in you for the last few days?

When you *know* your actual needs you are able to cater for them. If you do not cater for them, they get out of proportion and can be destructive.

Needs are closely related to motivation. Getting your needs fulfilled is an incentive: needs motivate you. In the manner in which you treat your needs lies the clue to what 'makes you tick'.

Rights

Rights, or fair claims, arise straight out of needs and are another of those bases for assertiveness. Rights are things we are entitled to. According to the Declaration of Independence of the United

States of America, we have the 'inalienable' right to 'life, liberty and the pursuit of happiness'. Seeing this in the light of assertiveness gives you kudos and certainty. Dickson (1982, pp. 29–36) lists 11 rights that a person has with regard to assertiveness. These are the rights:

- to state my own needs and set my own priorities as a person independent of any roles that I may assume in my life;
- to be treated with respect as an intelligent, capable and equal human being;
- to express my feelings;
- to express my opinions and values;
- to say 'yes' or 'no' for myself;
- to make mistakes;
- to change my mind;
- to say I don't understand;
- to ask for what I want;
- to decline responsibility for other people's problems;
- to deal with others without being dependent on them for approval.

Perls, the founder of Gestalt therapy, wrote this 'prayer' (1973, pp. 141–2).

I am I,
And you are you.
I'm not in this world to live up to your expectations.
And you're not in this world to live up to mine.
I is I.
And you is you.

Knowing and recognising your rights literally means knowing and recognising **boundaries**. In that way, you do not step on the rights of other people, and they do not step on yours: you are preventing them from stepping on your boundaries. Your responsibility is for yourself and *your* problems, not for others.

Many people find it very difficult to distinguish between their own and other people's boundaries. We think we are responsible *for* others when in fact we are responsible *to* them. This is why the notion of advocacy can be delicate: are we advocating our own needs or those of our clients?

You might like to repeat the Gestalt prayer and memorise it. It might come in useful in times of stress or conflict, or even when having to make a decision of whether to interiorise a feeling or make it explicit.

Wants

Wants are strong feelings and are often confused with needs or rights. Advertising is making us aware of many 'needs' that are basically wants. Do you need a new computer, to buy a particular book, or to have that operation?

We hear much said these days about rights, and most of these 'rights' are really egoistic wants. We are used to the idea that when we turn a switch, we will get light; in the same way, we think that our needs should be satisfied. When considering assertive behaviour, we need to be sure that we know the difference between needs and wants.

As a nurse, you may *want* many things that could improve your lot and that of your patients. You may have to weigh these against actual needs and possibilities, otherwise your assertiveness will only be criticised and ridiculed. To know clearly the difference between your desires and your needs may indeed be your most potent form of assertiveness.

Are you assertive?

Egan (1986, pp. 341–2) has outlined three 'Think Steps' for performing certain behaviours. Adapted to assertiveness, their essence is as follows:

At the *'Before' Think Step*, stop and ask yourself:

- Do I know what I need?
- Do I know what I am going to say about myself?
- Am I open (not prejudging a person or a situation)?
- Am I feeling sure of myself (not rejected)?

At the *'During' Think Step*, stop and ask yourself:

- Am I being myself (or what I think 'they' expect me to be)?
- Am I listening, trying to understand the other's point of view?
- Am I ready to accept some negative signs without letting them get me down, or blaming someone?
- I have a choice of how to deal with my feelings – am I ready to choose the better way?

At the *'After' Think Step*, stop and ask yourself:

- Am I letting myself get depressed that everything did not go perfectly?
- Is there anything I would like to add or say now?
- Is there anything I would like to question the other person about?

Advice on how to remain cool abounds:

- counting to ten;
- taking a few deep breaths;
- remembering your home telephone number;
- saying a prayer;
- thinking of the other person as an island – you sail right round it and only then land on it.

Such tactics give you space to become aware of yourself. They also give you the space to ask yourself:

- What is happening?
- What is the meaning of it?
- What am I going to do about it (see Chapter 2, p. 17)?

The areas in which being assertive is – or can be – difficult have been well outlined by Bond (1986, pp. 104–5) and are hinted at in the Think Steps. They are mainly to do with:

- making a request;
- saying no;
- making a point;
- setting limits;
- giving feedback;
- responding to feedback.

Below are assertive statements relating to each of the above topics. Make your own assertive remark for each, taking a situation that is familiar to you:

- *Making a request*: 'I need you to come now; this is not a matter for wait-and-see.'
- *Saying no*: 'No thank you, I don't want to buy any more tickets now.'
- *Making a point*: 'I find your explanation fascinating. You have, however, not answered my question.'
- *Setting limits*: 'Yes, this is my free weekend, and I want it for myself this time.'
- *Giving feedback*: 'You are really good at giving injections; I feel better just because you have given it to me.'
- *Responding to feedback*: 'You spotted that mistake rightly, but I don't agree with you that I make it all the time.'

The following is a set of aggressive, manipulative and (generally) non-assertive statements. Try making the same point in an assertive way:

- 'You make me so angry; no wonder I shout at you.'
- 'We have a no-smoking policy here; can't you see the signs?'
- 'Mind your own business. Who told you to teach me my own job?'
- 'You never seem to learn how to listen.'

Harassment

Many women experience men overstepping their boundaries as **sexual harassment**. Nurses have long been aware of this problem. Nurses are still too often depicted as sexual objects by the media. Patients and male colleagues making passes at female nurses, pinching a thigh or a bottom, or slipping a hand up a dress are all too common. Dickson (1982, p. 111) says that to say 'Stop it!' firmly may be in place, but it is often not enough.

Emma	Emma was a slightly older nursing student at a university where Simon was a lecturer. He had been assigned to Emma as her personal tutor. He took his role seriously and supervised Emma closely. Increasingly, he asked her to come for extra sessions as she needed help, he assured her. She was not convinced of this need. During the sessions he concentrated on personal issues, not academic achievement. When Simon asked Emma to see him in his office after hours she began to be seriously concerned. She wondered how long she had to tolerate this before it could be described as sexual harassment. (Tschudin, 1994, pp. 66–7)

Dickson (1982, p. 64) details three levels in which feelings can be expressed and says that these are particularly relevant in situations of sexual harassment:

1. Notice the feeling and acknowledge what is going on. The feelings at this stage may be of outrage or incomprehension, but they may also be of fear and a sense of being trapped. Trusting the intuition may be useful at this level.
2. Express the feeling verbally. A simple command of 'No' or 'Stop it' may be useful. It may be that a quick slap on the hand may be more effective. The problem is that this may be wrongly interpreted or may even be seen as physical assault.
3. The physical release of feelings through tears, shouting or trembling. This may be what Emma might have done, telling a friend or confidante about her situation. Once this has happened, it is also clear that more action is necessary, such as bringing the matter to the attention of someone who can do something about it.

Sexual harassment is not exclusively a women's problem. Men suffer equally from harassment, caused by both women and men. While it has taken a long time for the problem to be acknowledged by women, it is taking still more time for it also to be seen as a problem for men. Perhaps men have more frequently experienced harassment in other forms, only slowly recognising that sexual harassment is also part of their lives.

Other well-known forms of harassment are **bullying** and **victimisation**. They may not be immediately recognised as such, but when they are noticed, they must be stopped. **Racial harass-ment** is another form of discrimination, which is too easily present without being challenged (Cohen, 1992, p. 92). There are many possible ways of tackling these forms of abuse: Field (1996) mentions over 80.

Assertiveness is not really difficult – in fact, it is surprisingly easy. When you have been assertive a few times, you come to value yourself much more, feel in charge and respect yourself, and that makes you respect others. Your whole network of rela-tionships changes to one of confidence. This gives **courage** and invites **trust** and **honesty**. Once you feel less trapped in a role, doing things this way because you have always done them this way, you also release others from *their* traps. Assertiveness is putting into practice what you believe and value about yourself and others.

Assertiveness in nurses is often equated with patient advo-cacy (see Chapter 2). To speak up for the patient is indeed good, and nurses have too often in the past *not* spoken up for various reasons, fear being the most cogent. However, a nurse can only do this if she or he has been given permission by the patient. If the nurse takes on this task without permission, this is stepping on the patient's rights. Speaking up for patients means first of all speaking *with* them, hearing their story, values and motives.

Stress comes from many different directions. One way of dealing with stress is acknowledging it and learning to cope with the areas or relationships that are stressful. This takes assertive-ness. Above all, it takes courage: the courage of one's convictions.

References

Bond, M. (1986) *Stress and Self-Awareness: A Guide for Nurses*. London: Heinemann.

Cohen, P. (1992) 'It's racism what dunnit: hidden narratives in theories of racism', in Donald, J. and Rattansi, A. (eds) *'Race', Culture and Differ-ence*. London: Sage and Open University, pp. 62–103.

Dickson, A. (1982) *A Woman in Your Own Right*. London: Quartet Books.

Egan, G. (1977) *You and Me*. Monterey, CA: Brooks/Cole.

Egan, G. (1986) *The Skilled Helper*, 3rd edn. Monterey, CA: Brooks/Cole.

Field, T. (1996) *Bully in Sight; How to Predict, Resist, Challenge and Combat Workplace Bullying*. London: Success Unlimited.

Handy, C. (1997) *The Hungry Spirit*. London: Hutchinson.

Harris, T.A. (1973) *I'm OK – You're OK*. London: Pan Books.

Perls, F. (1973) *The Gestalt Approach and Eye Witness to Therapy*. New York: Bantam Books.

Tschudin, V. (1989) *Beginning with Empathy: A Learner's Handbook*. Edinburgh: Churchill Livingstone.

Tschudin, V. (1994) *Deciding Ethically: A Practical Approach to Nursing Challenges*. London: Baillière Tindall.

Chapter 5   Stressing yourself

Stress and stressors

If people say they are stressed or exhibit stress symptoms, they should be believed. What *feels* real has a basis in reality. (McNeel, 1987, p. 268)

Phrases like 'Pull yourself together', 'You shouldn't get involved' and 'If you think *you've* got a problem, just look at *my* workload' are heard far too often in nursing. And tolerated.

The basis of assertiveness and of any management of yourself is **listening** to yourself, to others and to the environment. Only by listening do you actually hear what is happening. Without knowing what is going on, you cannot change anything; you are deaf. And how often *are* we deaf, or do not believe what we hear. When we do not hear and believe what others tell us about themselves, our deafness is a danger to their lives.

Stress

What exactly *is* **stress**? The now famous definition of stress by Selye (1976, p. 74) is 'a non-specific response of the body to any demand, whether it is caused by, or results in, pleasant or unpleasant conditions'.

Stress is non-specific; everyone reacts differently and has different signs. That is why stress is so difficult to pin down and why people who are experiencing it are so often not believed.

Many theories and models have been created to describe and quantify stress (Stewart, 1992; Sheng, 1995). Dillon's (1983) descriptive five stages of stress are used here:

- *Stage 1: The honeymoon* Stress challenges you.
- *Stage 2: Fuel shortage* You have a vague sense of loss.

Challenge and enthusiasm have waned. You experience job dissatisfaction, fatigue, sleep disturbances and escape activities.

- *Stage 3: Chronic symptoms* Physical illness and loss of control of your emotions are recognised by you and by others.
- *Stage 4: Crisis* Your acid stomach becomes a bleeding ulcer. You become obsessed with your symptoms. Discontent becomes disillusion.
- *Stage 5: Hitting the wall* You lose control of your life. Without help from others you may never regain that control.

It may be interesting to compare these stages with some of the topics discussed in this book:

- Stage 1 and Stage 2 have to do with motivation.
- Stage 3 could fit in with the non-assertive behaviours.
- Stage 4 and Stage 5 link in with the description of the people coming downstream, about to drown.
- Stage 5 may be the point at which – with help – a person is able to discover the meaning of his or her life and return to the 'honeymoon stage', where life becomes challenging again. Sadly, that help is all too often lacking in nursing (but see Chapter 6 for strategies of support).

Stress is a necessary factor for survival, but where it leads to an excessive demand on an individual and is beyond his or her ability to cope, stress becomes destructive. The result of too much stress is a person's total inability to function effectively.

In the early stages of stress, the physical symptoms are the most obvious signs that something is amiss. Common coping mechanisms come into play, such as:

- being tired and sleepy;
- overeating;
- drinking;
- heavy smoking;
- uncalled-for aggression;
- withdrawing.

> ● Do you recognise any of these signs in yourself?
> ● Are these signs there all the time or only at particular moments?

It has been said that reading and learning about stress *gives* you stress where before you had coped very well! On the other hand, it may also give you insights into unrecognised aspects of stress, which can be helpful. Be aware of both possibilities.

With the physical signs go also the emotional aspects of stress:

● feeling useless;
● feeling incompetent;
● being touchy and irritable;
● having outbursts of anger;
● finding it hard to concentrate;
● weeping for no reason;
● experiencing violent mood swings;
● having feelings of panic;
● being unable to make decisions;
● being bored with oneself;
● having feelings of 'unreality';
● losing one's mind;
● becoming obsessive;
● having feelings of guilt;
● being impatient;
● having no more compassion;
● being forgetful and blocking;
● being unable to give attention to details;
● being prone to accidents;
● being irritable;
● being insensitive to others.

Some people try to compensate for these feelings and work twice as hard, showing everybody that they *are* competent and *can* cope. In that way, they feel less guilty. When this happens, they really are on the treadmill. The sad fact is that only an outside source can stop it.

Laura

Laura was a community nurse with long experience. Recently, one of her colleagues had been on holiday and another on maternity leave. This meant that Laura had the workload of three people. For the past two years, they had been short of a nurse as well, already adding to the caseload. Laura's paperwork got behind: she liked talking to patients better than writing about it. At the last yearly assessment, her manager had pointed out to her that she needed to be more careful with her records. She had tried, but she could not get enthusiastic about it. A new patient last week needed an injection, and Laura was aware that she had made a mistake in the dosage, but she told no-one. She made an extra visit to the patient, just to reassure herself, and he seemed all right. Then came the day when she nearly had an accident as she was driving far too fast on a small road, trying to get just one more visit in. When a phone call came from the office to say that another patient had complained that she had not visited her last week, she began to be worried. How did she forget? She checked in her diary and saw that she had ticked the appointment, meaning that she had been there. But she could not remember anything about the visit or the reason for ticking the appointment. To crown it all, she had now mislaid a box of controlled drugs and she needed to get them to a patient. The pharmacist would not give her another set without reason. The next day, she found the drugs in the home of another patient and realised that he had injected himself with them by mistake. She needed to see her manager urgently.

Think of yourself here.

- Do you recognise any of these signs in yourself?
- How long have they been there?
- Do you recognise them in others?
- What do you do when you meet them in yourself and others?
- How often do you feel indispensable?
- Do you feel personally responsible for the destinies of others?

Remember the Gestalt 'prayer' (see Chapter 4).

Before looking at ways of dealing with stress, it will be helpful to look more closely at the actual causes of stress. While most of us experience pressure, caused by others and by ourselves, this is normally temporary. The experience of pressure and stress can both be positive motivators, but only stress can lead to long-term problems.

Stressors

Stressors, the causes of stress, mobilize the body's fight/flight system to combat a perceived enemy. Chemical, physical and psychological changes come into play, preparing the body for a potentially life-threatening situation. (Stewart, 1992, p. 91)

When you listen to yourself, to others and to the environment, you realise that these three areas also form the three main sources of stress.

Stress from the environment

The **nursing culture** as it exists in Britain has much to answer for in creating stress. The image of the 'handmaid' is disappearing, but slowly. The mere fact that so many nurses want to learn about assertiveness shows that they feel they are not coping.

The image of the nurse who always carries out orders and never asks 'Why?' is not such a caricature. A few years ago, we were grappling with 'the unpopular patient': the patient who asked too many questions. We have had to accept that more and more patients these days do not simply say 'yes' and 'no' as appropriate, but nursing is having difficulty in accepting 'the unpopular nurse' – the nurse who asks 'Why?'

Routine has been the hallmark of this culture. This was outlined clearly by Menzies (1960) in her well-known study. Routine and the *status quo* protected student nurses in particular from 'getting involved' and from stress. Or so it was thought. Menzies showed that, on the contrary, these *led* to stress: relationships once formed could not develop; work begun could not be followed through; and, most revealingly, taking no part in decision-making rendered nurses cold and uncaring. From the outline of the temperaments in Chapter 1, it can be seen that perceiving people, that is, people who do not like routine but who respond to the immediate surroundings, tend to make good nurses.

- How much do you like routine?
- Does it help you or stress you?
- Were you aware that routine, deadlines and doing things by the book might be stressors?
- Acknowledge any insights and be aware of the meanings they have for you.

If the workplace culture promotes stress, so also does nurse education. The **pressure to succeed** is very strong. In the classroom, it is easy to portray nursing in an idealistic light, and all around, the pressure is on for more qualifications and higher degrees. This pressure is necessary when looked at from the point of view of the work and its demands. When seen from the standpoint of individual nurses, however, the pressure may be too intense, and nurses need to be able to say 'no' and not feel guilty about it.

Nurses often experience **guilt** when their **expectations** of themselves and those put onto them by others do not match up. The theory–practice gap is a thorny problem that will not go away. Tasks learned in the classroom will be carried out differently by the bedside, and admonitions of the importance of this and that are brushed aside in practice. Assurances about supervision and mentors ring hollow when learner nurses are left in charge when they have hardly learned how to *spell* 'haemorrhage' let alone met one.

However, not only the practical aspects cause stress. Nurses are required to give holistic care and be advocates of patients, leaders of teams, agents of change, responsible and accountable for their actions. Such ideals may not be achievable unless you know yourself well – your strengths and needs, your values and your boundaries, and where and when to enjoy yourself.

Work does tend to be the main stressor for people, but all sorts of factors connected with modern living also cause stress:

- commuting to work;
- housing and living problems;
- visits to the dentist and hospital;
- constant noise when quiet is required;

- the lack of pleasant excitement;
- emergencies and accidents.

You might like to add your own environmental stressors to this list and thus become more aware of your surroundings and what they mean to you.

Stress caused by other people

To start again with the nursing culture, there is a strange *cruelty* pervading the profession. '*I* was thrown in at the deep end, so I will make sure that I throw *you* in at the deep end' seems to be a perverse perpetuation of the culture. The lack of support from superiors for subordinates is sadly endemic. It seems that what causes stress and burn-out most quickly is not hard work, rotten hours and low pay but a *lack of positive enforcers* – of a 'thank you', of support and of the chance to have the need for self-actualisation fulfilled.

People who are *responsible for the destinies of others* are under greater occupational stress than are people responsible for managing material assets. 'Paper-pushing' may be stressful, but it does not usually involve having to make life and death decisions on a daily basis. It is usually the more sensing and feeling people who choose nursing, so it is not difficult to see that it is these very people who will suffer and get hurt in the process.

There has been a great deal of research into what stresses nurses most. A synthesis of some of them (Albrecht, 1982; Seuntjens, 1982; Hingley and Harris, 1986; Adey, 1987; Downey *et al.*, 1995; Heuer *et al.*, 1996) appears below.

> Look at the list, add your own stressors and perhaps number the items in order of your own priorities:
>
> - work overload;
> - staff shortage;
> - inadequate staffing;
> - the death of a liked patient;
> - the unnecessary prolongation of life;
> - unexplained changes; *(cont'd)*

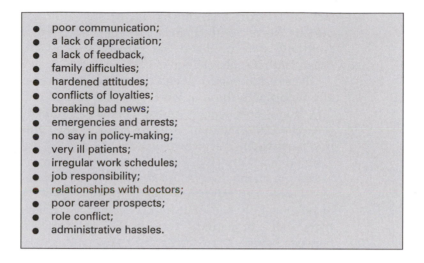

- poor communication;
- a lack of appreciation;
- a lack of feedback,
- family difficulties;
- hardened attitudes;
- conflicts of loyalties;
- breaking bad news;
- emergencies and arrests;
- no say in policy-making;
- very ill patients;
- irregular work schedules;
- job responsibility;
- relationships with doctors;
- poor career prospects;
- role conflict;
- administrative hassles.

This list shows clearly that the majority of stressors for nurses do not arise in the work *per se* but in the many *relationships* with other people involved with the work. Yet this is not so extraordinary, since most difficulties in life are caused by relationship difficulties. The problem of **conflicts of loyalties** cannot be overestimated. Too often nurses are 'piggy in the middle'. When it has been decided that a patient should not know his or her diagnosis, it is the nurses who have the most delicate job; when a drug error has been made, it is the nurse who gets disciplined; when a policy is not carried out, it is the nurse who bears the brunt.

Clause 13 of the UKCC *Code of Professional Conduct* (1992) states that 'in the exercise of your professional accountability [you] must… report to an appropriate person or authority where it appears that the health or safety of colleagues is at risk, as such circumstances may compromise standards of practice and care'. But when is a concern nothing more than snooping, and what happens when the appropriate person or authority is neither appropriate nor authoritative in action? The notion of whistle-blowing, or at least how to make concerns known and effectively dealt with (see Chapter 2), is as relevant here as in every sphere of professional life.

All these phenomena are not peculiar to nursing: most people know similar types of stressors. What *is* peculiar to nursing is the lack of support and care. It is therefore not surprising that nursing has one of the highest rates of suicide (Health Education Authority, 1988, p. 9) and that 'nurses top the list of psychiatric outpatient referrals' (Hingley, 1984).

The stresses caused by and through other people in life generally tie up with those of work. It is not possible to separate life into 'home' and 'work' – indeed, people who try to make them separate *add* to their stress, as in that way they split themselves into parts when everywhere else the trend is towards holism.

Bond and Kilty (1982) describe the stresses from other people as coming mainly from a *'bad atmosphere, inappropriate expectations* or *demands*, and *rejection*, or *not being understood'*. An awareness of other people and of their needs, and the ability to listen to them, will – or should – considerably reduce the stress created between people.

- What stressors act on you? Are other people responsible for these?
- What stressors act on others? Are you responsible for those?
- Are you aware of your needs?
- Are you aware of the needs of those who work with you?
- *When* are you most stressed?

Stress from within the self

There is much legitimate stress coming at us from outside ourselves over which we have no control. Simply, the way in which life is lived and organised is stressful. However, besides that, we ourselves put a lot of stress on ourselves, some of it willingly, some unwillingly, some quite unconsciously. The expression 'personal luggage' is a very apt metaphor for this aspect of life. Here are some of the issues that go into this luggage:

- expectations from childhood carried over into adulthood (see Transactional Analysis in Chapter 4);
- unresolved bereavements;
- guilt feelings;
- old resentments, now irrelevant;
- out-of-place ambitions;

- assumptions about others and self;
- perfectionism;
- not daring to succeed;
- feelings of dependence on others;
- not knowing when, where or how to say no;
- the inability to learn from one's mistakes;
- a fear of illness, loss of control;
- a lack of confidence;
- fear caused by memories of life events;
- oversensitivity to ideas and influences;
- a sense of not having a right to be here;
- unresolved relationships, particularly with family;
- overcaring for others.

When looking at the meaning of a situation or relationship, we may come across these things and they can block us. They each arrived there for a reason, but that reason no longer exists. Yet we still hang on to this luggage.

We cannot look at what stresses us without at some stage looking at these personal pieces of luggage.

- Do you recognise any of these items as yours? Perhaps mark them with different colours according to their importance.
- Why might these points be important to you?
- How much would you need to invest in emotional energy to resolve any one item?
- Are you ready to do that?
- If not, why not?

Just be aware of your choice; don't give yourself a hard time over it.

These items and questions bring us back to awareness, the temperament, the shadow, values, motivations and ways of asserting ourselves. However, it brings us back to these elements at a deeper level. To understand yourself at this level, you will probably need help.

As long as you were able to blame someone else – parents, the boss, the environment, 'they' – you were not responsible for your actions, nor for mistakes and failures from the past. When you look into yourself at the level of the stress produced from within yourself, you begin to see that the responsibility lies with you and within you, but it takes a lot of personal strength to accept this, cope with it and use it positively.

Responsibility is a delicate issue. As we learn to take responsibility for ourselves and our actions, we learn also *not* to take responsibility for others. Many caring people have unclear boundaries and therefore tend to 'take over'. They are the 'mother hen' types, the people with wide arms who can smother others. This, sadly, is not care for others but care for oneself, or selfishness: it is stepping on other people's rights.

Learning to care and to be responsible means above all learning to be **empathic**: going alongside, caring, being a companion, giving **freedom**. A true responsibility grows out of freedom, and freedom leads to rightful responsibility.

However, such insights and learning are almost impossible on one's own. As they concern relationships with others, these things have to be learned in company with others, often in groups. Some of the means of support outlined in the next chapter may be of use to you. This is also part of reflective learning and practice. But before that, some more points about stress have to be addressed.

Coping with stress

There are as many strategies for coping with stress as there are reasons for stress or responses to stress. Overall, there are two main approaches to dealing with stress:

- changing yourself and your attitudes;
- changing or removing the cause of stress.

Changing yourself

When you change yourself and your attitude, you do not change the cause of the stress, but you do not allow it to hurt you any more. Another prayer may be appropriate here:

God grant me the serenity
to accept the things I cannot change;
courage to change the things I can;
and wisdom to know the difference.   (Niebuhr)

Self-awareness means taking the time to sit down with your-self to listen to the parts of yourself that hurt and are tense and stressed. There are many practical ways in which this awareness can be reached:

- relaxation;
- meditation;
- listening to music;
- chanting a mantra;
- praying;
- journal writing;
- imaginative drawing;
- visualisation/fantasy journeys;
- writing poetry.

One of the difficulties is that a stressed person usually has a short concentration span, and for any strategy to work, it has to be continued. To give up after one or two attempts is defeatist. Miracles do not just happen: we have to work at them. It may therefore be helpful to do some of those exercises with the support of another person or a group.

- Which of these ways is the most accessible one for you?
- It may help to find a friend who has similar inclinations.

Changing or removing the cause of stress

This is the real uphill work. The work you have already done on motivation and on assertiveness will form the basis of it, as will your values.

As a simple outline of the management of any change, the four steps of the nursing process form a good framework:

- assessment
- planning
- implementation
- evaluation.

Any strategy for change has to take into consideration:

- what has gone before;
- what is the present reason for the change;
- what is hoped for and expected from the change.

It will need to include the questions:

- What is happening?
- What is the meaning of it?
- What is the goal?

It will also need to take into consideration:

- memories
- dreams
- associations.

Each of these questions and items corresponds roughly to the equivalent stage of the nursing process. Evaluation should not just be tagged on at the end as an afterthought; it should go on throughout the process in the form of feedback and revision.

Maritta

Maritta was a Finnish nurse working in Britain. She told Jason, a colleague, about her difficult relationship with her mother. Maritta went home only about once a year, but it was enough to make Maritta dread her trip home.

It was now a few weeks before she was booked to fly home. She asked Jason to help her work on a strategy for coping with her relationship, at least for the duration of the holiday. They considered the items and questions above. Maritta decided that her best option would be not to allow an argument to develop, and instead of getting upset, she would not allow herself to mind when her mother made a remark that would normally hurt.

(cont'd)

> Although they did have their differences, Maritta's decision meant that she did not get angry, and the inevitable contretemps did not poison the atmosphere. On her return, she realised that she had actually enjoyed her holiday! Although this tactic did not solve the problem of the relationship, it made the atmosphere easier, and that was a good enough goal for the present. She thanked Jason for his help and later asked him to work more with her to enable her to understand the relationship with her mother better.

When you know your needs, wants and possibilities, you can begin to establish goals. When you know where you are heading, you are free of the many unnecessary distractions that encumber your life and tend to drag you down. When you are working towards realistic goals, you have become a round peg in a round hole and have stopped trying to fit into someone else's (or your own) fabricated square.

Pot-Mees (1987) has outlined certain things that nurses should be and do in order to succeed without stress:

- be true to oneself;
- have realistic expectations;
- consider one's own feelings as important.

Solving a problem in these circumstances may not seem as impossible as you had imagined.

Positive stress

One way of dealing with stress is actually to counter it with stress that gives you a 'high'. Here are some suggestions:

- competition/sport/physical activity;
- directly confronting difficulties;
- decorating a room;
- preparing and having a party;
- giving yourself a treat;
- doing something you would not normally do;
- giving yourself time out.

After having taken some practical – and possibly distracting – step, you may be able to face a particular problem in a new, and perhaps unexpected, way.

You might also like to try the following exercise:

- Isolate your problem as clearly as you can. Then imagine that you are in the ideal world, without any constraints. You could be what you are and do what you like best doing.
  - Where would you be?
  - What would you be doing?
  - Who would you be with?
- Take these questions seriously. Don't just *think* about them; let your imagination roam. Your fantasies are free – let them come and delight you.
- When you have seen yourself in fantasy without constraints, imagine now all the constraints that could possibly be put upon you:
  - What constraints are there upon you?
  - What constraints do you put upon yourself?
  - Who stands in your way and prevents you from being yourself?
  - Who/what is the agent that constrains you?
  - What is the message of this constraint?
  - What is the value for you of such constraints?
- Think about these constraints, and take them seriously; they may be able to show you the goal towards which you have been working but which you have not recognised, or the goal which could realistically be attained.
- When you have thought about these issues, write them down, and perhaps ask a friend or counsellor to help you to formulate a goal.

Imagination is not simply kids' stuff. It is the greatest faculty we have for seeing possibilities. It is also, for adults, the single most underused resource for moving forward. Trust your imagination, and use it to help you find your blind spots. When you have identified those, you are in a position to deal with them, and in this way move forward; when you can name something, you have a hold over it.

There are clearly many more aspects to stress than are mentioned here. In a climate where more and more is expected of people, perhaps the two most difficult words to say are 'yes' and 'no': no to stress and yes to life.

References

Adey, C. (1987) 'Stress – who cares?' *Nursing Times* **83**(4): 52–3.

Albrecht, T.L. (1982) 'What job stress means for the staff nurse.' *Nursing Administration Quarterly* **7**(1): 1–11.

Bond, M. and Kilty, J. (1982) *Practical Methods of Dealing with Stress.* Guildford University: Human Potential Research Project.

Dillon, A. (1983) 'Reducing your stress.' *Nursing Life* **3**(3): 17–24.

Downey, V., Bengiamin, M., Heuer, L. and Juhl, N. (1995) 'Dying babies and associated stress in NICU nurses.' *Neonatal Network* **14**(1): 41–5.

Health Education Authority (1988) *Stress in the Public Sector; Nurses, Police, Social Workers and Teachers.* HEA.

Heuer, L., Bengiamin, M., Downey, V.W. and Imler, N.J. (1996) 'Neonatal intensive care nurse stressors: an American study.' *British Journal of Nursing* **5**(18): 1126–30.

Hingley, P. (1984) 'The human face of nursing.' *Nursing Mirror* **159**(21): 19–22.

Hingley, P. and Harris, P. (1986) 'Burn-out at senior level.' *Nursing Times* **82**(31): 28–9.

McNeel, B.T. (1987) 'Stress', in Campbell, A.V. (ed.) *A Dictionary of Pastoral Care.* London: SPCK, p. 268.

Menzies, E.P. (1960) 'A case-study in the functioning of social systems as a defence against anxiety.' *Human Relations* **13**: 95–121.

Pot-Mees, C. (1987) 'Beating the burn-out.' *Nursing Times* **83**(30): 33–5.

Selye, H. (1976) *The Stress of Life,* 2nd edn. New York: McGraw-Hill, p. 74.

Seuntjens, A.D. (1982) 'Burnout in nursing – what it is and how to prevent it.' *Nursing Administration Quarterly* **7**(1): 12–19.

Sheng, R.H. (1995) 'Stress and adaptation' in Heath, H. (ed.) *Foundations in Nursing Theory and Practice.* London: C.V. Mosby, pp. 195–207.

Stewart, W. (1992) *An A–Z of Counselling Theory and Practice.* London: Chapman & Hall.

UKCC (1992) *Code of Professional Conduct,* 3rd edn. London: UKCC.

Chapter 6　Supporting yourself

Support

If I am not for myself
Who is for me;
and being for my own self
What am I?
If not now, when?　(Hillel 'the Elder', 70 BC–AD 10)

Support for nurses has long been declared an 'urgent top prior-ity' (Briggs, 1972), but nothing much has happened to put this into practice. Sadly, more and more nurses are coming down the river about to drown.

Lorinda

> Lorinda was a young sister on a surgical ward. Her father had died three months previously after a long illness. Her line manager, who had been very supportive, was about to move to another job. To crown it all, Lorinda then had a miscarriage. She felt that this at least she could not share with her colleagues, but she was often 'scatterbrained' and seemed distracted. Her GP gave her a few days off, calling it stress. She confided in a friend, who suggested that they go together to a newly formed women's group. There Lorinda began to realise that she was not alone with her feelings. The leader of the group suggested to Lorinda that she should also see a counsellor from CRUSE, the bereavement organisation, and gave her a name. Lorinda felt hesitant at first but then took up the offer. After a few times of meeting, she could understand her feelings and reactions better and was able to face the world again.

Support is many things. Each person needs different types of support, depending on temperament, work environment and so on. Support is anything that:

- affirms you;
- encourages you;
- helps you to be creative;
- helps you to come to deeper insights about yourself and your life;
- helps you to fulfil your potential;
- helps you to have realistic goals in your life and keep working towards them;
- helps you to change goals, particularly during and after a time of crisis;
- challenges you.

> Stop for a moment and look at this list. Which area do you think is most applicable to you at the moment? Do you recognise anything of Lorinda within you? If you do, make a note of it.

In an ideal setting, the employing authority would ensure that the necessary support was available to all staff. Employers have both a responsibility to their staff to see that they come to no harm (Hancock, 1983; Tschudin, 1985) and an interest in *keeping* staff, because experienced staff are valuable and because turnover and absenteeism are very costly. All the same, neither self-interest nor legal requirements have as yet led many employers to provide adequate emotional support. If you want support, therefore, you have to go and get it. What you want badly enough, you will get. What is good enough to have is worth fighting for.

Managers will often say, 'They can always come and talk to me' or 'The occupational health department staff have counselling facilities' or 'If they want a group, they can have one.' But this is not good enough. 'A chat' with the line manager is not always appropriate, and most occupational health departments are geared towards rehabilitation, advice and guidance rather than professional counselling. Setting up an effective support group needs expertise and commitment.

Four different possibilities of support are outlined here. You may find that you need others and that many others are available. You may then have to go and get them. Keep in mind, however, that what works for one person and one area may not work for another person or another area. You need to find the support that is appropriate for you.

Professional and practice development

To achieve job satisfaction and prevent 'burn-out' and 'drop-out', a nurse must be self-directing and must maintain control over her own practice. (Hickey, 1982)

This sums up quite neatly many of the things said in this book so far. One of the pillars of 'practice' is **education**. Post-registration Education and Practice (PREP) gives clear enough guidelines of the statutory needs involved, but this is only the minimum and it is not very much. To have **job satisfaction**, you also need **personal satisfaction**, and that may involve learning about and expertise in the aspects listed.

Interpersonal skills
● Interviewing skills;
● Group/team leadership skills;
● Supportive skills (particularly for and with dying patients and their relatives);
● Committee/chairmanship skills;
● One-to-one helping and counselling skills;
● Assertiveness skills;
● Personal defence skills;
● Recognition and management of stress.

Training and teaching in ethical issues
● Knowledge of ethical and moral language and principles;
● The UKCC *Code of Professional Conduct* (1992) and related guidelines;
● Issues such as professionalism, advocacy, informed consent, accountability, confidentiality and responsibility.

Management and assessment skills
● Management of a ward/unit;
● Management of a budget;

- Safety aspects;
- Management of time and resources;
- Assessment of learner nurses;
- Assessment of health care assistants;
- Assessment of volunteers.

Have you had any education in any of these areas? Which, do you think, is the most important area in which you now need more training? Make a list of your priorities:

- Find the course you need (in the nursing press, through personnel officers or through enquiring at training establishments, for example).
- What is your *goal* in doing such a course?
- What do you *want* from such a course?
- What is your strategy when approaching your manager?
- How can you be working towards getting what *you* want rather than what *he or she* wants from you?
- What stress will be involved?
- Who will support you emotionally in your approach (if the course is long or expensive, or both), during the course and after a possible rejection of your request?

As an exercise in assertiveness, you might like to think how to approach your manager to sponsor you to go on a course of your choice to learn the particular skill you need.

Preceptors

Every newly qualified nurse should have a period of about four months under the guidance of a preceptor to make the transition from learner to staff nurse smoother. Maben (1996) found that, in her research, half the nurses interviewed had no such help, and the other half had very good help. As always, an idea can work well somewhere and not so well elsewhere. The *reality shock* that many nurses experience should never be underestimated, and even when someone is coping well, a **mentor** is invaluable. Indeed, the concept should ideally include all staff, everybody having a recognised person who is concerned with the well-being of a colleague.

Counsellors

The British Association for Counselling states that 'the overall aim of counselling is to provide an opportunity for the client to work towards living in a more satisfying and resourceful way' (BAC, 1990). All too often in nursing, 'counselling' is equated with disciplining. Because of that, nurses hesitate to make contact with a counsellor, or do not know what to expect if and when they meet one.

It is often a crisis, a point of recognition that 'I cannot cope any more', which brings a person to a counsellor. At such a time, however, it is impossible to think straight, feel clearly, get in touch with emotions and memories or look to some future satisfying living. What the person (client) needs is to be heard, to feel accepted rather than judged and to be given support in whatever way is appropriate to cope with the next few hours or days. Only after that can the real work of counselling and development begin.

The concept of this book – managing yourself – is precisely what **counselling** is about: to enable you to get to know yourself, your strengths and needs, to find motives for your values, to find meaning and potential for living and to have the ability to put this into practice.

In a counselling situation, the presenting problem is very often not what eventually turns out to be the main focus. The main focus is the *person*, your way of being and doing, and this can occasionally take quite some time to come to terms with. The strengths and needs, the temperament and the shadow are often reluctant to reveal themselves.

Because each person is so different, it is almost impossible to say either what goes on in counselling or what counselling should be or could help you with. The more aware you are of yourself, your strengths, your needs and your failings, the easier counselling might be – or the more demanding and challenging.

If you are looking for a counsellor or a counselling service, you should always assure yourself of certain points:

● Is it *professional*? Is the counsellor trained, to what standard and in what mode or theory? People who have done a two-day course may not be able to deal with the personal material that may emerge during a session.

- Is it *confidential*? Is no-one going to know about your visits unless you tell them?
- Is it *independent*? To whom is the counsellor accountable? This may be important if there is a fear that reports may be used for assessment or promotion.

It has been said that counselling is 'for better or for worse'. A counsellor can be an effective 'midwife', so that the client can solve his or her own problems, form his or her own goals and adjust his or her style of living. However, an ineffective counsellor may not be able to handle such situations well.

Much *helping* is done quite incidentally in daily life: it is often invaluable and quite adequate. This, however, is not counselling but making use of some of the *skills* of counselling.

Support groups

Support groups are perennial discussion points because of their regular appearance and disappearance. Nurses often want to set them up but then do not have the know-how or incentive to keep them going.

Support groups will only be effective if they are action-orientated. As such, they should deal with issues of professional identity, techniques for stress management and methods of conflict management. When they do this, they also increase staff members' sense of self-esteem and self-confidence while increasing their knowledge of and skills with the dynamics of relationships.

Within such a framework, support groups are very variable. They may:

- have one goal;
- have several goals;
- meet weekly;
- meet monthly;
- have a leader;
- take turns at leadership;
- meet for a set number of occasions;
- be ongoing;
- be for nurses only;

- be interdisciplinary;
- be for nurses of one grade only;
- be for all staff on a unit/ward;
- be a time for relaxation and sharing;
- have a fixed agenda;
- be small;
- be large.

The main reason why groups are often difficult to maintain is the lack of basic preparation. The most important – and least often asked – questions are those given in Chapter 2:

1. 'What is happening?' Nurses are always quick to find solutions, and a support group may be a 'solution' to a particular situation, but the problem may not have been well enough analysed.
2. 'What is the meaning of it?' What is the underlying or hidden reason why a group is needed at this moment and for this group of people? When this becomes clear, the rest becomes clear too.
3. 'What is your purpose or goal?' This may be any of the items just mentioned or some other, but unless that purpose is clear to all participants, a support group remains a talking shop. An important element is that the group, its aims and purpose are and will be regularly evaluated by all participants.

The National Association for Staff Support (NASS) in the health services has excellent guides and packs for setting up and running staff support groups. The address is given at the end of the chapter.

How are you supporting yourself?

Throughout this book, I have been asking you to be aware of yourself, your thoughts, feelings, motives and needs, and to note them down. This was done to enable you to gather your energies and focus them to help you manage yourself more effectively – more resourcefully and more satisfyingly.

The quote at the beginning of this chapter:

If I am not for myself
Who is for me;
and being for my own self
What am I?
If not now, when?

could be an ideal starting point for a personal philosophy, an 'aims and objectives' for your life, or for writing your personal set of principles.

If you want to get anywhere, you have to have a plan, a strategy. You need to know the how, who, where, what and why of a thing or situation before you can be a part of it or tackle it.

Much of life is a constant striving for control. Humankind's survival depends so much on the individual's ability to live with the environment. This is not so much a domination of others (I'm OK – you're not OK) as a co-operation with and adaptation to the given situation (I'm OK – you're OK). This takes effort, and the stress produced in the process is considerable – unless you know what you can and cannot do, and what the difference is.

As a part of what this book can give you, I would therefore like to invite you to work out your personal philosophy and make that a part – even the basis – of the way in which you manage yourself. The following questions and exercises are suggestions in formulating such a philosophy. If you have better, or other, questions and means, please use them.

- What is good in your life at this time? Make a list and find as many things as possible.

- What is difficult in your life at present? Make a list of the items you recognise, or refer to your notes of earlier exercises.

- What do you recognise as weak or undeveloped characteristics?

- What do you recognise as particular needs?

- What life events have formed you most? In what ways? Be as specific as you can.
  What has changed for you after such (an) event(s)?

(cont'd)

- Who are you when you are alone?

- What three things about your life do you value most?
  If you could have just one value, which one would you choose?
  Study your motives for choosing this one, and note it down.

- What do you like most about your colleagues? your friends? your family?
  What do you think they like most about you?

- What do you like *least* about them? You cannot change them, you can only change yourself and your attitudes to them. What change might you want or need to make?

- What meaning is there for you in the relationship with a close person (name the person)?

- What meaning is there for you in the relationship with a person (name him or her) with whom you do not get on but with whom you cannot avoid contact?

- What motives keep you wanting to help other people? Do you help them, or do you help yourself?
  Empathy is said to be the ability to get close to a person while keeping one foot on firm ground in order to help that person objectively. What is your firm ground in helping?

- When things go wrong, do you blame *them* (the things) or *someone*? Do you blame yourself? How much responsibility do you take for unfortunate circumstances in your life?

- Do you recognise any particular needs that you have at the moment, but have not yet mentioned? Think about them, then note them down.
  Check with the diagram on page 42 to see in which category your needs are. Are they all in one or in different categories? What do you deduce from this about yourself?

One person's personal philosophy statement runs like this:

I am I.
I am responsible for myself.
When I feel myself responsible for others I take away their freedom.
When they take away my freedom, I am diminished.

Therefore I have to say no, not defiantly, but creatively, for myself and to
  them.
When I am lonely I tend to use others for my own ends.
When I know my firm ground it gives me comfort, strength and joy. Only
  I can cultivate my own ground.
Others are my friends in so far as I am a friend to them. I cannot expect
  them to give of themselves. When they do, it is beautiful.
I can will, and strive, and yet I may not succeed. Having done all, and not
  succeeded, I will accept what is given, and not regret.
When I know my limits of strength, courage, empathy, and go as far as
  those limits but not beyond them, I am wise.
Wisdom teaches me to extend my limits ever wider in patience,
  goodness, and respect. I can and will accept the challenge.

(Mäder, 1988; translated and adapted)

This is how one person has formulated the main ideas of the
meaning of her life. She felt it necessary to make it clear to
herself that she has the responsibility for her own actions. She is
helping herself in order to help others. This example may give
you some hints about the kind of things you would like to say
about yourself.

The last two points in the statement quoted may sound contra-
dictory. This is deliberate. A statement of philosophy is a guide, a
map, an indicator of the limit or boundary of yourself and your
world. But you are not 'bound' by such a document. Self-awareness has a 'growing edge', and from time to time the statement
has to be rewritten and adapted. It is not a tablet of stone.

Some people have collections of quotes and wise sayings that
they use to reorient themselves when necessary. Some people
make little notes and put them in places where they see them
frequently in the course of the day. They become the significant
statement for the time being and sum up a philosophy or direct
the mind towards new ideas or goals. Perhaps you also have
such means of reorienting yourself.

Sometimes it feels as if self-awareness is a never-ending and
painful digging up of more and more skeletons, and you may
sometimes wish you had never started on this whole business.
This is perhaps when a note, your personal statement of intent or
philosophy may come in useful. Looking back every now and
again to where you have come from is very encouraging. Seeing

how you have developed and grown in insight, wisdom and ability can be the most affirming thing you do for yourself.

Supporting yourself is looking after yourself. When you know your self, your strengths and needs, you are comfortable with yourself – comfortable enough to go beyond yourself and help and care for others in such a way that they are enhanced rather than dominated, freed to be creative themselves rather than being dependent. This is why support is so important: it helps you to become yourself, and through that, others become themselves.

References

Briggs Report (1972) *Report of the Committee on Nursing*. London: HMSO.

British Association for Counselling (1990) *Code of Ethics and Practice for Counsellors*. Rugby: BAC.

Hancock, C. (1983) 'The need for support.' *Nursing Times* **79**(38): 43–5.

Hickey, J.V. (1982) 'Combating "burn-out" by developing a theoretical framework.' *Journal of Neurosurgical Nursing* **14**(22): 103–7.

Maben, J. (1996) 'Preceptorship and support for staff: the good and the bad.' *Nursing Times* **92**(51): 35–8.

Mäder, D. (1988) Personal communication.

Tschudin, V. (1985) *Ethics and Management of Support for Nursing Staff*. North East London Polytechnic: unpublished BSc (Hons) dissertation.

Useful address

NASS (National Association for Staff Support) 9 Caradon Close, Woking, Surrey GU21 3DU.

Chapter 7 Celebrating yourself

Celebrating

> Those who are able to celebrate life can prevent the temptation to search for clean joy or clean sorrow. Life is not wrapped in cellophane and protected against all infections. (Nouwen, 1978, p. 95)

By celebrating, I do not mean the sort of ceremony when you put on a gown and mortar board and have your photo taken. As awareness exists only in order to go beyond it, so **celebrating** means celebrating yourself and celebrating the other person. How, you may ask, does this relate to managing yourself?

Self-awareness comes into its own when the awareness of others is authentic, liberating and creative. You manage yourself well in relation to others; you manage others well in so far as you manage yourself well. This means finding a balance between work and play, personal and professional life. It means that you see and acknowledge what you have and may find that it is enough. We shall 'never cease from exploration', but we need to stop and see again and again what it is that we have explored.

The three elements of past, present and future that I have repeatedly used can also be applied to celebration. I would like to start with the present, with affirming, before going on to look at the other elements of celebrating, namely remembering and expecting.

Affirming

Celebrating is **affirming** yourself and affirming life. However, like awareness, this is, for two reasons, not easy to do these days.

77

First, celebrating means taking time, but the world is in a hurry: a sense of breathlessness pervades all we do. An advert is only valid if it states that the job is for this 'busy' ward or centre. A meal is not a time for rest and company but a mere stop for refuelling. Always rushing about means never affirming anything. Always looking for more and better means simply getting there faster. But where?

Second, the opposite is also true: those who do not rush about stay asleep. These are the armies who cannot be bothered, who find anything an effort. They give you the impression that one day they will not even know the difference between a wedding and a funeral.

Both by rushing about and by being asleep, we have largely forgotten how to celebrate. We generally celebrate only good things; by bringing 'bad' things into awareness, we 'celebrate' them also. Staying with the good and the bad for a while gives us insight. Because we do not celebrate the 'bad' things, we do not learn from them. We put up heroes and leaders and imagine that their qualities will do the work for us.

As a first step in affirming yourself, stop and think:

- Who are the three people, living or dead, whom you admire most? Write down their names.
- Who are your heroes? Write down their names.
- What are the qualities for which you admire them?
- When you have thought about this last question, try to recognise those same qualities in yourself.

Affirming yourself gives you confidence and satisfaction and the ability to evaluate yourself. When you know yourself, your strengths and your needs, you are less tempted to seek approval from others – which might well be only flattery anyway.

When you know who you are or what you are, you do not need to wear a mask or look for status or authority. When you know yourself and are sure of it, you are an **authentic** person.

Then you can say with all simplicity, 'That is what I do best, and that is what gives me satisfaction.'

Self-awareness and self-knowledge give you a **freedom** to be yourself and express yourself in appropriate and easy ways. Freedom is the real reason for this celebration.

Miriam

> Miriam is a senior nurse in an intensive care unit in a European capital. She is also an official guide in her city. Every week she works four days as a nurse and one day as a guide.

Peter

> Peter is a psychiatric nurse with an interest in wildlife. He is a ranger in a national park where he can satisfy his hobby.

Maintaining the sense of affirmation and freedom is not easy. **Power** and **authority** can creep up surreptitiously, and selfishness then abuses that power. This is why celebrating is not an ego trip. It is done in order to become more authentic, more real, more open.

When you are affirmed – by yourself and by others – you can affirm others. It is usually in moments of crisis, doubt or failure that someone needs to be affirmed most. When you have failed in some way – real or imaginary – you do not need to be told, 'Serves you right'. You need to have someone there who asks, 'What happened? Tell me, I'm here to listen.' When you know what it felt like for you, you have a good idea what it may feel like for others. You can make use of your experience, both of the crisis and the resolution of it, to help others. This is **empathy**. Being there does not mean taking over. The difference between effective and ineffective help lies here: giving attention gives the other room to grow; taking over is a selfish act. Affirming is respecting the person and respecting his or her freedom; taking over is abusing this freedom.

Rogers (1980, p. 143) has described empathy as being not only a skill but 'a way of being', and Roach (1984, p. 2) has described caring as 'a total way of being'. 'Getting involved' with another is inevitable, in fact, it is the only possibility. This is when the boundaries become unclear and the edges blurred. In doing that, however, each recognises the humanity of the other. They are not helper and helped any more, but each helps the other. That is when the edges begin to 'grow'.

Respecting the other also means not judging that person, or any way of life, action, situation or view, until you have heard the story about it. It is so easy to make assumptions, to jump to conclusions, to finish a sentence for the other. That is taking over and assuming a responsibility that we have not been given. We affirm others only when we hear *their* story. Respecting the other helps him or her to grow and be creative. In respecting, you are respected. In creating, you are created. Some people have called this co-creativeness – an apt term for this kind of work.

This leads to being **supportive**. It does not mean checking up on the other but 'being alongside' as the person finds his or her own way:

People don't like to be 'should' upon. They'd rather discover than be told. (Dass and Gorman, 1985, p. 157)

When we 'should' on others, we take away their freedom. Another person's freedom is her or his basic right. When we take it away, we diminish our own freedom.

Supporting is helping others in every way to complete their work of creating. It may mean challenging them to wake up, or challenging them to slow down. Whatever it is, it is a being alongside while they find *their* goal, *their* purpose of life, themselves and their actions.

That can only be done with a great deal of **hopefulness**. Those who prefer to sleep tend to be afraid of the future; those who rush about have no sense of the past. The truth lies in the middle, in the present. To come to that middle, that authentic way of being, is hard work, with many trials and failures. If we believe that another person is worthy of being affirmed, we need the hope to support her or him not just to a goal, but also on the path to that goal.

- When was the last time you were affirmed by someone?
- Who was the person who affirmed you?
- When did you last affirm someone?
- What was your reason for doing so?
- What did *you* gain by affirming another person?
- How might you affirm yourself now?
- Why not do it right now?

Remembering

When there is no **memory**, there is nothing to celebrate. We can only stand in the present because of the past from which we have come. The reason for rushing about is often to forget, to eradicate and to make believe it never happened.

Other people give their memories power to destroy them. In the film *The Life That's Left*, a family is shown in which one of the young sons has been killed in an accident. His mother has kept his room just as he left it. The other members of the family are no longer to laugh at home: there is literally a deathly hush all over the house. The memories gradually destroy the family as a whole and the individuals in it.

Memories are 'the stuff of life'. To live life to the full, we have to *hear* our own and other people's memories:

most people here [in the nursing home]… they just want to tell their story. That's what they have to give, don't you see? And it's a precious thing to them. It's their life they want to give. You'd think people would understand what it means to us… to give our lives in a story.

So we listen to each other. Most of what goes on here is people listening to each other's stories. People who work here consider that to be… filling time. If only they knew. If *they'd* just take a minute to listen! (Dass and Gorman, 1985, pp. 112–13)

We each have our story to tell. Before that, we each have our story to *make*. We are responsible in large part for what we do with our lives and ourselves.

- If you were to write your autobiography, what highlights – which memories – would you choose for an outline?
- Choose any one particular memory and stay with it. Is it a good memory or a difficult one? Simply be aware of it and of your choice: don't judge it.
- In what way has this memory shaped your present – that is, in what way are you still celebrating the memory?

Memories are important aspects of our lives. **Traditions** in families and nations keep a wider memory alive for the future. Religions keep sacred memories and memorials, and celebrate them regularly. In order to be what we are, we have to realise where we have come from.

The best things in life – family, friends, health, nature – come free, and we are therefore inclined to think that we have a right to them. Yet they are not ours to *keep* but to *treasure*. To take them for granted is to overlook their intrinsic worth.

Celebrating by remembering is 'counting the blessings', seeing the good, the noteworthy and the advantages.

On page 30, I asked what keeps you in nursing. The answer you gave then is relevant here: celebrating the memory shapes your present and your future.

Give yourself permission to celebrate your successes. Such celebration is the basis of your professional confidence.

Our celebrating of memories allows us to help others to celebrate theirs. Self-awareness is fulfilled when it leads to helping others come to new insights, new celebrations.

When you have been with a person and affirmed her or him, there comes a time when you need to look inwards. In order to discover the *meaning* of a situation, an event or life, you need to see it in the perspectives of your memories. Has anything like this happened before? What was the outcome? What does this remind you of? The memories then lead to associations with the present, and that is the raw material for finding a goal to move forward.

| Jill | Jill's daughter had only lived for three days. Every year on her birthday, Jill busied herself making Christmas puddings, giving herself a lot of work so as not to have time to think. This ritual was repeated for 16 years. In that year she had learned a 'therapeutic technique' and was able to explore her emotions. In doing so she was able to get in touch with the past in a way which she had not done before. This seemed a very simple step, but one so profound that when the day of her daughter's death came round again, she did not make Christmas puddings but treated herself to a very expensive bouquet of flowers, wept and felt a little subdued but also very peaceful. (Tschudin, 1996, p. 37) |

Memories from the past often come suddenly into focus. Associations can be made which, to an outsider, might not make much sense, but which to the person concerned are (literally) of vital importance.

When these memories are brought into the present, acknowledged, 'counted' one by one and given the necessary attention, the whole person is affirmed.

> ● What are your significant memories?
>
> Perhaps write them down and keep them alive for a few days, being thankful for how they have enriched your life: celebrate the memories.

Expecting

We can look back only because we have a sense of the future. It may seem a contradiction in terms to say that we need to celebrate the future. Only in the dictionary does success come before work...

We celebrate the future by taking seriously our ability to create it.

Neither the sleepers nor the rushers have much of a sense of the future. Without a sense of where you are going, you are not getting anywhere. This is why it is so important to have goals, or a sense of meaning, in life; without them, people drift here and there – both physically and emotionally.

Throughout the reading of this book, you have looked at yourself. In thinking about your own meaning and your own philosophy of life, you have prepared the way for celebrating your future. The next chapter should help you to put this into practice, at least in a professional way.

When you have experienced the need for some goal, meaning or direction in life, you can also help others to come to similar insights.

- What are you expecting from your life?
- What do you hope it will give you?
- What are you prepared to give to life?

By celebrating what you expect, you are also celebrating those as yet unknown or undeveloped parts of yourself: the shadow. The shadow is part of you, longing to be acknowledged. Some parts of it will always remain hidden, but the areas that have been revealed in and through the memories and associations ask to be taken seriously and dealt with. This is, indeed, where celebrating the expectations comes in: by not being afraid and thereby restricting the future. **Fear** inhibits so much growth. Celebrating the future is a kind of celebrating of the abandonment of fear.

'Giacomond'

I was given a card of a painting by Quint Buchholz entitled 'Giacomond'. The picture shows a small part of very steep roof against a night sky with a full but watery moon. From the gable runs a rope into the air on which a man stands with one foot. The other foot is in the air. The man is pulling the rope up and holding it loosely in his outstretched hands.

This picture is a wonderful image of stepping out, unafraid, into the night and the dark. Every step into the future is into the dark, on an unsupported rope. It is impossible – yet it is the only way forward. What is dark will eventually become light, although it may not be the light we expected. What is impossible will eventually become possible, although perhaps differently from how we expected, because we have dared to step out.

Discovering a meaning in life, setting yourself a goal or describing your purpose, often opens up a wide vista. To come to an insight, exclaiming 'I see', is really to see into the future. This is like the step into the air. It is that essential step from the present fixed and heavy shell around us into the future and a more satisfactory way of being.

Alice and Rowan	Alice and Rowan were in their late fifties. They had not been able to have children and had suffered all their lives because of this. As their nieces and nephews grew up, they took a lively interest in *their* families. They were godparents of Annabel and helped with great interest to organise her wedding. When, a few years later, Annabel told them that she and James could not have children either, the two couples sat for a long time together, crying and being aware of each other's pain and what this had meant for each of them. It was James, Annabel's husband, who said finally, 'You've helped me to understand what suffering is about.' This seemed quite incredible to Alice and Rowan, who had only felt pain. They looked at each other and tears started again. But this time they were tears of joy. Annabel and James had given them the gift of themselves, and beyond their pain they seemed to be falling in love all over again. They could have no children, but they had each other to cherish. Their old age suddenly seemed like a new life.

- Do you remember the last time when you had an *aha!* experience? How did it happen? What has changed for you since that experience?
- Stay with the experience as you remember it, and see how it has brought you forward. Have you taken it for granted, or are you grateful for it? How?

To stand with another person at the point of expecting the future, 'dreaming' about it and seeing possibilities is to be present at one of the most exciting moments that life can offer. I have talked in terms of helping someone; in truth, it is not so much 'helping' someone else as enabling another to become what she or he already is. You are not so much a helper as a 'midwife' to an experience. In that role, you are not only helping another: you are fulfilling yourself.

Rogers (1978, p. 92) describes well what this means:

I have found my greatest reward in being able to say 'I made it possible for this person to be and achieve something he could not have been or achieved before'. In short I gain a great deal of satisfaction in being a facilitator of becoming.

You might like to think of – remember – a similar time or experience when you have been with someone, perhaps agonising for a long time before coming to a conclusion, a goal, a decision or an insight. When that moment came, the other was helped, but you were affirmed in your own person too.

● What was the turning point?
● What memories do you have of it?
● In what way can these memories now help you? In what way are you, or should you be, celebrating them?

'Celebrating' in an authentic way is going back to awareness and seeing it from a new angle. *Awareness* is looking at yourself from 'outside'; *celebrating* is looking at yourself from 'inside', from experience. Awareness is knowing what 'strokes' you give to others and they give to you, and how and when you give and receive them. Celebrating is living them, but they are not simply strokes any more: empathy – caring – has become a way of life.

This is what managing yourself is about: being with others in such a way that both you and they are freed, liberated, moved forward. When you manage yourself, you celebrate yourself and those around you.

We are made up of memories, experiences and hurts that have wounded us and that we have allowed to wound us, but such wounds need not rule our lives. If we can allow the scars to form, the wounds ask us to go beyond them, into the future, to acknowledge their potential for us to become wounded healers. That is celebration.

References

Dass, Ram and Gorman, P. (1985) *How Can I Help?* London: Rider.
Nouwen, H.J.M. (1978) *Creative Ministry*. New York: Image Books.
Roach, M.S. (1984) *Caring: The Human Mode of Being, Implications for Nursing*. Perspectives in Caring Monograph 1. Toronto: University of Toronto.
Rogers, C. (1978) *On Personal Power*. London: Constable, p. 92.
Rogers, C. (1980) *A Way of Being*. Boston, MA: Houghton Mifflin.
Tschudin, V. (1996) *Counselling for Loss and Bereavement*. London: Baillière Tindall.

Chapter 8 Developing yourself and your career

NB The term 'practitioner' is used in the text to refer collectively to nurses, midwives and health visitors, that is, all registered nurses.

A nursing or midwifery qualification that results in registration on a part of the UKCC Register for Nurses, Midwives and Health Visitors is a great achievement for every individual. For most of us who embark on a nursing or midwifery career, the challenges of that initial programme of study are great as the demands of being a student, learning in practice placements and preparing for professional practice impact on every aspect of our lives. Expectations are high – clinically, academically and professionally – from those influencing and responsible for the programmes, and students often feel great pressure during their three or four years of study as they prepare for registration.

Professional development

A central feature of most preregistration programmes is the need for students to 'know themselves' – to gain insight into their own value systems and to understand their feelings, prejudices, coping mechanisms and emotions, for example about issues and situations they meet in practice and which impact on how they influence patient care. Perhaps one area in which concentration on personal perspectives would be as beneficial is that associated with the factors influencing the individual's ability to develop professionally. This chapter aims to devote attention to how you, as an individual nurse or midwife, may begin to influence, very positively, your professional development and professional choices. To a great extent, the impetus for developing yourself professionally is to work actively towards the assessment and understanding of the career opportunities that exist following registration.

When you qualify in your chosen field of practice, you face an ever-increasing range of work and career opportunities. Initially, your choices may be influenced by the availability of posts and by pressure from a variety of sources to gain certain experience. Nevertheless, the choices you make in your career are just as important as those made later on. Registration is an initial step, and if you wish to progress in clinical practice and in any other aspect of nursing or midwifery practice, experience, further study, the maintenance of a professional portfolio and additional clinical qualifications are usually essential. There follow details and suggestions about how to make effective career-related decisions that will impact on your own professional development.

In recent years, career patterns and opportunities for nurses and midwives have changed in response to the clinical grading structure, introduced in the late 1980s, the English National Board (ENB) Framework for Continuing Professional Education and the Higher Award (ENB, 1991a), the UKCC recommendations for Post-Registration Education and Practice (PREP: UKCC, 1997) and *The Scope of Professional Practice* (UKCC, 1992a). Also, the range of roles for nurses, in particular, is increasing alongside changes in titles bestowed on nurses working in practice settings. This is particularly so in the hospital sector; for example, 'team leader' is replacing 'sister' as a job title in some settings, and others such as 'nurse practitioner' and 'clinical development nurse' are now commonplace.

Patterns of employment are also changing. Currently, 35 per cent of nurses working in the NHS work part time, this being the highest ever recorded figure. More nurses are opting for employment in the private sector and in nursing homes. In 1996, of the 640 000 registered nurses, 300 000 worked in the NHS. Table 8.1 illustrates the whole-time equivalents, by grade, and it can be seen that there are proportionately fewer posts at grades F, G, H and I compared with those at D and E. This bottleneck is bound to have implications for progression and career development, particularly between E and F grades.

Table 8.1 Total whole-time equivalent nursing posts in 1996

Whole-time equivalents	Scale
D	84 757
E	93 414
F	31 414
G	58 636
H	10 959
I	3 906

(Royal College of Nursing, 1996)

More employers appear to be recognising that they need to be able to accommodate the working needs of qualified staff, particularly women (who make up 90 per cent of the nursing workforce). As more women with dependants need to work, employers are beginning to respond by offering a greater range of part-time opportunities, including flexible rostering and promotion. In a study by Seccombe *et al.* (1993), it was found that 47 per cent of nurses take a career break, the most common reason being maternity leave. It was also found that 75 per cent of women working part time have family commitments, although they experienced negative effects on career progression opportunities. Male nurses, on the other hand, despite making up only 7 per cent of the workforce, occupy 14 per cent of the managerial posts (Seccombe *et al.*, 1993) and are less likely to have to adapt to a break in service.

Other studies have revealed attitudes to other important aspects of a nurse's working life. These include evidence that more nurses and midwives are working excess hours than they did in the 1980s, the main reason being sickness and absence cover, unexpected peaks in workload and staff shortages (Seccombe and Ball, 1992). In addition, 50 per cent of nurses in this study expressed concern about the levels of nursing care and nursing turnover rates (found to be highest among younger nurses), and overall disappointment was expressed about career prospects.

From these studies, some of the pressures and concerns have been revealed. In recent years, there have been examples of nurse redundancies. Nurses are also striving for more suitable hours of work and pay, and less stress in the workplace, which appear to influence the frequency of job changes (Seccombe and Ball, 1992).

The need for nurses to feel in control and to be proactive in the process of their own career management is as important now as it has ever been. The range of roles are illustrated in Table 8.2. In the light of this rather awesome choice, and the prerequisites needed to be eligible for such posts, it is now necessary to explore the strategies that you will need to adopt to plan your own career appropriately.

Table 8.2   Nursing and midwifery roles in a hospital setting

Remember that all posts are subject to satisfactory application, references, interview, health screening, registration on a part of the UKCC Register for Nurses, Midwives and Health Visitors and appropriate disclosure and assessment under the Rehabilitation of Offenders Act 1974

Post	Grade	Role specifications
Staff nurse Associate nurse Staff midwife	D	These are usually first posts following registration. Posts at this grade are often appropriate for nurses and midwives with no previous experience in a particular speciality
Senior staff nurse Primary nurse Staff midwife	E	Usually one year's experience in the speciality, qualification with an ENB 997/998 Teaching and Assessing course, experience of supervising and assessing students, and qualification with the associated ENB clinical course is expected. Evidence of personal and professional development, effective communication skills, competence in the field and potential leadership skills are expected
Ward sister Team leader	F/G	**The role of specifications for F grade posts will usually include:** • all the E grade specifications • a period of experience in the speciality (for example, 2 years) • evidence of the potential to lead a team • evidence of clinical and managerial skills
Clinical nurse specialist	G/H	**The role specifications for G grade posts will usually include:** • all the E and F grade specifications
Practice development nurse	G/H	• clinical experience in the speciality (for example, 3–5 years • evidence of advanced study, for example diploma or degree level in a subject relevant to the post • evidence of proven clinical, managerial and leadership skills

Table 8.2 continued

Post	Grade	Role specifications
Lecturer/practitioner	} G/H	• evidence of research ability and/or experience • the potential for innovative practice
Clinical nurse adviser	} G/H	**The role specifications for H grade posts will usually include:** • the G grade specifications • evidence of the experience of leadership qualities • the ability to advise and offer development support across a clinical directorate • the ability to work as a member of a management team • evidence of managerial, professional, research and clinical experience relevant to the post • the ability to initiate and respond to innovations, policies and quality initiatives

Table 8.3 Nursing and midwifery posts in the community

As well as the essential requirements needed for employment (as summarised in Table 8.2), most post-holders are expected to be car drivers.

Role	Grade	Qualification(s)	Role specifications
Staff nurse	D/E	RGN	Most staff nurse posts are aligned to district nurse teams as part preparation for secondment to a degree or diploma course leading to the registration as a district nurse. Applicants are usually expected to have 6 months–1 year staff nurse experience
Staff midwife/ Team midwife	E/F	RM	As team midwifery develops, more opportunities exist for midwives to practise in a range of settings in response to the need for the continuity of care of mothers. F grade posts usually require at least 1 years' experience and the ENB 997 course
District nurse/ Team leader (Community nurse in the home)	G	RGN (Part 1 or 2) DN Degree or Diploma	There is a range of full- and part-time posts for registered district nurses. District nurse team leaders are expected to have at least 2 years' experience as a district nurse, a teaching qualification (for example, ENB 998), leadership potential and managerial experience. They manage a caseload of patients

Table 8.3 continued

Role	Grade	Qualification(s)	Role specifications
Health visitor/ Primary health care nurse (Public health nurse)	G	RGN/RSCN HV degree or diploma	There are opportunities for full- and part-time posts. Health visitors are members of a primary health care team. Some posts specify that possession of the RSCN qualification is desirable or essential if specialist care of individuals in the 0–18 age group is required. They manage a caseload of patients
Community nurse	D/E	RGN RMN or RMNH RMN and RMNH Dip. Social Work (SW)	Staff nurse/community nurse are titles which are often used interchangeably (see above). There are a range of posts for those with RMN and/or RMNH qualifications, including day centres, homes for those with learning disabilities and/or physical disability, caring for the elderly mentally ill and rehabilitation. Experience of caring for children and adolescents is often desirable
Community psychiatric nurse (CPN)	E/F/G	RMN	At least 1 year's experience is expected and 2 is usual for F and G grade posts. Many posts offer opportunities to specialise, for example in substance misuse, eating disorders or psychotherapy. CPNs work within a multidisciplinary team and must be able to manage a caseload – these requirements are essential
Community paediatric nurse	E/F/G	RSCN (Part 8 or 15) DN degree or diploma, plus module(s) in community paediatric nursing	Currently few posts and courses exist for this specialist role
Team leader – mental health	G/H	RGN, RMN	A range of posts exists. The post-holder usually manages a team of nurses responsible for the care of mentally ill people in a range of health care settings. Skills and experience in community mental health care is usually essential

Table 8.3 continued

Role	Grade	Qualification(s)	Role specifications
School nurse		RGN or RSCN on Parts 1, 2, 8 or 15. ENB School Nursing course	Health monitoring and health education and promotion are the key aspects of this role, which is part of the community nursing service. Working closely with teachers
Practice nurse	E/F/G	RGN (Part 1 or 12). ENB Practice Nurse course (not essential)	Practice nurse posts vary greatly in terms of prerequisites and role criteria. A range of full- and part-time posts is available. Clinical experience in the acute sector is expected (usually 1–2 years). In-service education is often essential, as practice nurses are expected to undertake a range of activities not commonly practised in hospitals, for example health screening and immunisation
Occupational health nurse	G	RGN (Part 1 or 12). Occupational Health Nurse course (diploma)	Most occupational nurse posts exist outside the NHS. Opportunities abound in organisations, for example the leisure industry, multinationals, manufacturing and commerce. Posts often demand an occupational health qualification, as well as qualifications and experience in a range of health care settings. Effective management skills are essential as is the ability to operationalise necessary health care strategies and services among a workforce

Career pathways in nursing

Historically, the traditional career expectations of nurses and midwives would be to practise in a range of settings following registration. This may also have included undertaking a second course of study and, for nurses especially, to qualify on another part of the register before specialising in an aspect of clinical work. This would, in turn, lead a number of nurses and midwives into senior clinical posts, for example that of sister. Further options would lead many into posts (usually part time) so that family commitments could be met. For those remaining in practice, promotion would usually mean a move away from clinical practice to posts with either a managerial, educational or research emphasis.

Times and opportunities have changed. There are fluctuations in the job market as well as changes in the hierarchical management system that have been influenced by the clinical grading structure and the dissemination of managerial responsibilities to ward and unit level.

There is currently a national shortage of nurses, particularly in the high-dependency and mental health sectors, and recruitment into nursing is problematic, especially for the branches of learning disability and mental health nursing. As in previous years, this situation is likely to change and hopefully improve, particularly as the growth and development in community care services impacts on the nursing posts available and the employment prospects that follow.

Despite the current recruitment and retention patterns, there is a positive job market for nurses and midwives that is enhanced by the increased mobility of nurses, changes in the range of hospital- and community-based posts, and gradual improvements in opportunities for flexible and part-time contracts.

Nurses and midwives who register achieve both a professional and an academic qualification. There are expectations that they progress both clinically and academically for the majority of clinical posts beyond D grade (as illustrated in Tables 8.2 and 8.3).

A career pathway is the individual's own professional experience and is usually characterised by the development of clinical, academic and professional activities. Progressing through the clinical grades illustrates how experiences, skills and competencies are developed alongside educational and training demands to fulfil statutory and employment requirements. The chosen pathway may be characterised by a particular specialist field of care, for example neonatal intensive care, palliative care or elderly mental health care, as well as the dominant purpose of the role, for example management, research or education. It is with these latter details that we see significant changes in roles and responsibilities as, for example, clinical nurses and midwives face more and more managerial demands, nurse and midwife educators face the demands of academic life while needing to maintain clinical involvement, and nurse and midwife managers become more concerned with the impact, implications, costs and benefits of education, training and research.

As you develop your career, the quality of your working life is all-important. This quality may be influenced by:

● the need for job satisfaction;
● the need for job security;
● the need to develop responsibility within a role;
● the need for a supportive working environment;
● the need to develop both personally and professionally;
● the need for suitable working hours;
● the need for suitable travel facilities.

You will have your own priorities, but work commitment and stability are positively influenced by job satisfaction and a supportive working environment.

The traditional view that a career should involve promotion is not a central need for everyone. On the contrary, there are many nurses who experience great job satisfaction from long periods in a post, often over many years, and who do not choose to strive for the challenges of changing to a new field of practice or to seek promotion. A key factor for those remaining in clinical practice is that to pursue a pathway involving promotion may, in turn, distance them from practice. There are proportionately few senior clinical posts at G, H and I grades. However, those that do exist may carry with them extensive clinical and caseload responsibilities, for example as a stoma care sister, clinical nurse specialist for infection control or pain management, health visitor, community midwife or community psychiatric nurse. These examples illustrate how developments in clinical roles have facilitated expert practice alongside managerial and educational responsibilities.

One of the most significant challenges facing all nurses at the present time is the development, maintenance and control of clinical practice. The opportunities to acquire senior clinical roles is limited, although the UKCC (1994) is intent on exploring the implications of advanced nursing practice. It states:

Advanced nursing practice is concerned with adjusting to the boundaries for the development of future practice, pioneering and developing new roles responsive to changing needs and with advancing clinical practice, research and education to enrich professional practice as a whole. (UKCC, 1994, p. 20)

As clinical roles develop, you need to be mindful of your personal career pathway as well as your clinical career pathway. Manley (1997) recognises that advanced practice incorporates expert practice requiring nurses to integrate the roles of manager, educator and researcher – a tall order, but one which is observed in settings where senior nurses administer care and have responsibilities for the management of practice. This is particularly so in specialist clinical areas where the majority of the nursing workforce are registered nurses, in nursing development units and where the nursing culture recognises, practices and evaluates a reflective approach based on research-based practice.

Employers of nurses and midwives

The array of clinical posts available to nurses is extensive (see Tables 8.2 and 8.3 above). In addition to these are opportunities for those wishing to pursue posts with a nursing, midwifery or health visiting perspective but which may not have a major focus on those aspects of practice. Table 8.4 illustrates a range of these posts, and the associated employers, most of which assume previous practice experience and demand qualifications of a professional and academic nature and often extensive experience in activities relating to the role.

Table 8.4   Employers of nurses and midwives outside the NHS

Charitable organisations	For example, Macmillan Nurses
HM Armed Forces	• Army – Queen Alexandra's Royal Army Nursing Corps (QARANC) • Royal Air Force – Princess Mary's Air Force Nursing Service (PMAFNS) • Royal Navy – Queen Alexandra's Royal Navy Nursing Service (QARNNS)
Local authorities and social services	For example, care managers in residential homes

Table 8.4 continued

Nursing agencies	For example, opportunities for short- and long-term employment in a range of settings, some with international links
Occupational health services	For occupational health nursing posts in a range of workplace settings
Private hospitals	For a range of nursing and midwifery posts, and for enrolled nurses
Publishing houses	For example, those with a nursing/health care background and with suitable experience may find employment within the world of publishing in the health field
Prison Service nurses	With an RGN and RMN qualification, nurses may pursue a career caring for offenders, providing rehabilitation and supporting women with babies in special units
Statutory bodies	The UKCC and the National Boards for England, Scotland, Wales and Northern Ireland employ professional officers with specialist backgrounds in nursing, midwifery and health visiting as well as mental health and learning disabilities nursing. Applicants would normally have extensive professional, managerial or educational experience
Trade unions and professional organisations	Relatively few posts exist in organisations concerned with providing trade union and/or professional support for their members. For those with interests, for example, in policy development, employment law, trade union work and professional issues at a national and international level, this is worth exploring
Universities and colleges of further and higher education	Since the amalgamation of colleges and schools of nursing with higher education, teachers (that is, lecturers, senior lecturers and principal lecturers) of nursing, midwifery, child health, mental health and learning disability are based there and are concerned with pre- and post-registration education. Effective links with health authorities and Trusts remain, as do opportunities for research activities across the specialities

You need to be mindful of the implications of opting for employment outside the NHS and the impact on employment rights, contracts and contract renewal, as well as pension rights and continuing education and training opportunities. This is particularly important if you are considering working abroad as you will need to establish appropriate personal and professional insurance cover. The professional trade unions and statutory organisations, for example the Royal College of Nursing (International Department), the Royal College of Midwives and the UKCC (see Appendix), can be particularly helpful.

Making the most of career options and opportunities

It can be seen that the range of employment opportunities is overwhelming. For the newly qualified, particularly nurses, the choice is broad and to some extent reflects the range of experiences completed as part of the pre-registration programme. The range may be tempered by the number of vacancies and the suitability of posts (at D grade) for the newly qualified practitioner. For midwives, first posts tend to be available in hospital-based midwifery units. For registered nurses (adult branch), the range is great, particularly during periods of nursing staff shortage (see examples in Table 8.5). The most common first posts are offered in surgical and medical directorates and are still referred to as general surgical and general medical in nature despite the often specialist work undertaken in the acute sector. Some of these posts are rotational and have contracts of a year or more. Today, it is more common to find first posts being advertised in high-dependency and intensive therapy units. Likewise for RSCNs, hospital-based posts are common as first posts, and employers expect that general experience in paediatric, medicine or surgery will be undertaken before developing specialist skills in, for example, oncology, high-dependency care or nephrology.

Table 8.5   First posts for newly registered (adult branch) nurses – D grade staff nurses

General medicine
General surgery
Day case unit
High-dependency unit
Intensive care unit
Coronary care unit

RMNs usually face a wide range of choices, from acute psychiatry to elderly mental health care and rehabilitation. Learning disabilities (RNMH) nurses usually find D grade posts in hospital or community-based settings, for example assessment units and community homes, caring for people with a range of physical and learning disabilities.

First posts in primary health care settings are rare. Most community care managers prefer staff nurses to have had a period of hospital-based practice (usually 6–12 months) prior to a post with, for example, a district nurse team.

Opting for employment with a nursing agency or an NHS Trust 'bank' is a useful alternative for you if, at registration, you need some flexibility with your working pattern but perhaps need an income to sustain expenses in the short term. Although useful, employment with these agencies does not usually contribute positively to your career because there is a lack of control over where experience is gained. Also, supervision, preceptorship and educational opportunities are not usually provided, and the experience is often disjointed. However, agency and bank work are useful for subsidising other employment, for supporting educational endeavours and for maintaining clinical contact if opportunities for this do not exist within the terms of a full- or part-time post.

Bearing in mind the range of opportunities following registration, it is pertinent to examine factors influencing career options and professional development. These fall into three main categories as follows:

1. professional requirements;
2. personal and work needs;
3. family/social needs.

Each will be explored and discussed.

Professional requirements

All practising nurses, midwives and health visitors are subject to a range of professional and statutory requirements, all of which you should be familiar with, so the key components only are given here.

The UKCC sets standards for education, training and professional conduct through the application of the Nurses, Midwives and Health Visitors Acts of 1979 and 1992. *The Code of Professional Conduct for the Nurse, Midwife and Health Visitors* (UKCC, 1992b) and the UKCC *Guidelines for Professional Practice* (UKCC, 1996a) offer guidelines for the standards expected of all practitioners in terms of their responsibilities to the public.

Post-registration education and practice

The maintenance of effective registration
All practising nurses have a responsibility to develop and maintain their own professional knowledge and competence.

The UKCC states the following Post-Registration Education and Practice (PREP) requirements for maintaining registration (1997, p. 6):

- completing a notification of practice form at the point of re-registration every three years and/or when your area of professional practice changes to one where you will use a different registerable qualification
- a minimum of five days *or equivalent* of study activity every three years
- maintaining a personal professional profile containing details of your professional development
- a return to practice programme if you have not practised for a minimum of 750 hours or 100 working days in the five year period leading up to the renewal of your registration (from 1 April 2000).

The initiative to maintain these *minimal* standards lies with each individual, and employers often demand higher standards. All professionals have a responsibility to keep up to date, and nurses are no exception. This is not an exercise to be conducted in isolation from colleagues, peers and line managers; on the contrary, the management and co-ordination of any professional development activity needs to be conducted with the interests of patients, the practitioner, the team and the organisation in mind. The UKCC recognises a range of categories of study that are relevant to this process, including:

- new approaches to practice;
- research into aspects of practice;
- patient-centred initiatives;
- educational activities, personal study and literature reviews.

Notification to practice

To maintain your registration, you also have to complete a notification to practice form (UKCC, 1997, p. 8):

- every three years when you apply to renew your registration.
- if you change your area of practice to one where you will use a *different registerable qualification.*
- if you return to practice after a break of five years or more.

The personal professional profile

The UKCC has, since 1995, required all practitioners to maintain a personal professional profile. This document is a personal collection of written evidence of professional development, based on a 'regular process of reflection and recording, what you learn from everyday experiences, as well as planned learning activity' (UKCC, 1997, p. 13).

Students, during their preregistration courses, are now expected to maintain a professional profile, and the features for post-registration are very similar. The profile becomes a record of all aspects of professional activities, experiences, qualifications and reflections about work-related activities and professional developments. Table 8.6 provides you with a framework for developing your own profile, although you may wish to use a published work, for example the ENB portfolio (ENB, 1991b).

Table 8.6   Framework for developing a profile

The profile may be structured as follows:

Personal details	Full name Previous surname Title Date of birth Address for correspondence Personal index number (PIN)
Academic qualifications	Secondary school: subjects, grades, dates
Further/higher education	Qualifications, subjects, grades, dates
Professional registerable qualifications	For example, RGN, RM, RMN, RNMH, RSCN, EN(G) and the part of the register. Qualification, date, college of nursing/university department or faculty where obtained
Professional recordable qualifications	For example, National Board certificate courses or occupational health nursing. Qualifications, dates, college of nursing/university departments or faculties

Table 8.6 continued

Professional qualifications	For example, Diploma in Nursing. Qualifications, dates, college/university departments or faculties
Professional employment	Begin with your current post and then document these chronologically
Other relevant responsibilities	Here is the opportunity to list other activities in which you are involved; this may include: ● other previous employment, for example prior to commencing nursing course or voluntary work ● membership of professional organisations and interest groups ● research activities ● publications ● management activities, for example membership of committees and working parties
Record of education and formal learning activities	Give details of: ● courses, study days, conferences, seminars and workshops attended and visits to other centres ● personal learning activities undertaken, for example teaching activities and the use and application of literature/research relevant to your work The UKCC (1996b) advises that for each of these you need to give details of: ● its relevance to your professional practice; ● what you hope to achieve from it; ● your assessment of the outcomes of your activities; ● the time spent on each event and on any follow up work.
Record of working hours	Hours worked during the three year period should be recorded
Self-assessment and evaluation of performance have	This is your opportunity to comment on: ● your experiences to date and what and how you learned from them ● the contribution these experiences have made to your role and development as a registered nurse ● specific events that have occurred, to document them in detail on the basis that they were useful to you and what you learnt from them. These critical incidents may be positive or negative in outcome, for example breaking bad news, comforting a bereaved family or managing a ward for the first time ● your perceptions of your current skills and competencies and your needs for further development
Future planning	This is your opportunity to look ahead and document your plans and objectives for the future. Aim to have a few statements of intent that may, for example, relate to ideas concerning the development of a specialist skill or undertaking a course of study

The UKCC (1996b, p. 7) summarises the benefits of using a profile as follows:

- to help you assess your current standards of practice.
- to develop your analytical skills – these are fundamental to your professional practice and the profiling process will help to sharpen your ability to reflect constructively on and analyse what you do.
- to enable you to review and evaluate past experience and learning in order to plan your continuing education and career development.
- to provide effective up-to-date information for use in application forms and interviews when you apply for jobs or courses.
- to provide evidence of what you have learned from your own experience. This may allow you to obtain credit toward further qualifications from an institution of higher education through schemes such as APEL (accreditation of prior experiential learning) and CATS (credit accumulation and transfer system).

Your professional profile is your personal record. It must be maintained and up to date. It is probable that you will be asked to submit it to an interview panel when you are interviewed for a professional post.

These professional requirements exist to promote and maintain standards of practice, so educational opportunities exist to support this process, in particular in relation to ongoing professional education.

The PREP initiatives commenced in 1991, and there have, since then, been significant developments in terms of supporting the education and professional development of practitioners. The original notion behind PREP was to ensure a continuum of professional development for all nurses, midwives and health visitors in practice.

Preceptorship was established as a means of providing support for newly qualified practitioners during the first four months following registration. Preceptors support, guide, teach and facilitate in a way that should enable the development of competence, confidence and skills. After an initial period of six months in a first post, applications are often made to undertake National Board clinical or specialist courses, usually lasting six months, in order to gain a recordable qualification. The choice of courses is very broad and places are often limited, so competition is high. (Table 8.7 illustrates a range of popular courses.) The courses can be undertaken as stand-alone qualifications and can also be taken as part of a diploma or degree programme. Your local department of continuing nursing education within a university, school or faculty will advise you of the local provision. The National Boards also provide details of the location of these courses for their respective country (see Appendix).

Table 8.7   A range of popular courses

Examples of English National Board courses of particular interest to RGNs, for example adult branch nurses:

- Accident and Emergency Nursing – ENB 199, No. 3
- Altered Body Image – A58
- Breast Care – ENB A11, No. 9
- Burns and Plastic Surgery Nursing – ENB 264, A15
- Cardio-thoracic Nursing – ENB 160, 249, A13
- Complementary Therapy – A49
- General Intensive Care – ENB 100
- Gynaecological Nursing – ENB 225
- Haematology and Bone Marrow Transplant – N14
- Infection Control Nursing – ENB 329, 910, N26
- Infection Control and Wound Management – N54
- Maxillo Facial Nursing – A15
- Neuromedical and Neurosurgical Nursing – ENB 148, N42
- Oncology Nursing – ENB A27, 237, 285
- Ophthalmology Nursing – ENB 346, N76
- Orthopaedic Nursing – ENB 219
- Pain Management – N53
- Perioperative Care – A21, N33
- Practice Nursing – A51
- Renal and Urological Nursing – ENB 136
- Renal Transplant – N39
- Research – ENB 850
- Stoma Care – ENB 216, 980
- Surgical Nursing – A25
- Teaching and Assessing – ENB 998
- Trauma Care – N52
- Wound Management, Tissue Viability – N49

Examples of English National Board courses of particular interest to:

Midwives   For example:
- Teaching and Assessing – ENB 997
- Accountable Practitioner – A26
- Accountable Practice – A31, N70, N68, N66
- Women Centred Care – N67
- Neonatal, Advanced Practitioner – A19
- Neonatal Intensive Care – ENB 405, 904

Table 8.7 continued

Learning disabilities nurses	For example: ● Learning Disability Nursing/Mental Handicap – N59 ● Abuse of Adults – N65 ● Advances in Behaviour Modification – ENB 705, 937 ● Community – ENB 740, 806, 807, 939 ● Challenging Behaviour – N02 ● Mental Handicap (Child) – ENB 958 ● Multiple Handicap/Child – N43, 972 ● Physical Disability, Rehabilitation – ENB 913 ● Sensory Handicap – N16 ● Services and Support – A63
Children's nurses	For example: ● Acutely Ill – A37 ● Child Protection – ENB 430, 970 ● Community Paediatrics – A50 ● Paediatric Intensive Care – ENB 415 ● Managing Pain – N51 ● Oncology – ENB 240 ● Renal – ENB 147 ● Respiratory Disorders – A64
Mental health nurses	For example: ● Acute Psychiatric Nursing – A61 ● Behaviour Modification – ENB 705, 937, A28 ● Child and Adolescent – ENB 603, 975, A03 ● Community – A66, A16, ENB 811, 812, 989, 992, 993 ● Elderly – A39 ● Enduring Mental Health Problems – A60 ● Forensic – N30, N56, A71 ● Rehabilitation – ENB 655, 945 ● Therapeutic – A68

Courses numbered 100–870 and with a prefix A: 40 days or more, recordable qualification.
Courses numbered 901–998 with prefix N: less than 40 days, ENB award.

Along with PREP and the professional, statutory requirements (previously described) is the ENB framework for continuing education and the ENB Higher Award, which features the ten key characteristics for professional practice. These have been embraced by many nursing and midwifery degree level courses in ENB-approved institutions from across the country. They are as follows (ENB, 1991b):

1. professional accountability and responsibility;
2. clinical expertise with a specific client group;

3. use of research to plan, implement and evaluate strategies to improve care;
4. team-working and building and multidisciplinary team leadership;
5. flexible and innovative approaches to care;
6. the use of health promotion strategies;
7. facilitating and assessing development in others;
8. handling information and making informed clinical decisions;
9. setting standards and evaluating quality and care;
10. initiating, managing and evaluating clinical change.

Embarking on the Higher Award as part of a course of degree-level study involves a tripartite arrangement between you as a practising nurse, midwife or health visitor, your manager and the lecturers with the responsibility for the course, within a university. You can negotiate your route through the course, which is usually part time, following successful application and the establishment of a learning contract. The maintenance of your professional portfolio is part of the process as it facilitates the recording of the achievement of the ten characteristics.

Credit Accumulation and Transfer Schemes (CATS)
There is an expectation that academic qualifications are now an integral part of the standards expected of all practitioners. Today, nurses and midwives undertake a diploma-level course as part of their preregistration programme; the rest achieve a degree. CATS points are academic currency for academic achievement at certificate, diploma and degree level, as illustrated in Table 8.8. Therefore, achieving a diploma gives you 240 points, a degree 360 points.

Table 8.8   Credit Accumulation and Transfer Scheme (CATS)

CATS level 1	Certificate level	120 credits
CATS level 2	Diploma level	120 credits (240 points accumulated)
CATS level 3	Degree level (honours)	120 credits (360 points accumulated)

If, as a diplomate, you apply for a diploma or degree course following registration, and the course has themes similar to those previously studied, your CATS points may allow you to be exempted from aspects of the course, for example a module. Not only are previous academic achievements assessed and valued, but so too are previous experiences.

Assessment of prior learning (APL) and assessment of prior experiential learning (APEL) are complex systems for giving credit for previously formed learning experiences (APL) and professional and clinical achievements (APEL) towards another qualification. When you apply for a course, the process of application will incorporate these perspectives and will usually involve a detailed assessment of previous experiences, formal interview and scrutiny of your portfolio.

All statutory preregistration and midwifery courses, and those subject to National Board approval, are subject to conjoint validation, for example academic and professional validation usually to CATS level 2 or 3.

ENB careers network facility

To assist with the process of clarifying professional requirements, the ENB has a careers network facility that focuses on post-registration opportunities (Table 8.9). This facility also involves a local network, and the ENB has a register of senior nurses and lecturers who are available to give local advice (the ENB careers office and your local nursing and midwifery department within the university should be able to advise you).

Master's level qualifications

There are some posts for which Master's level qualifications are desirable, if not essential. These include lecturing posts and senior research and management posts within universities, Trusts and professional and statutory organisations. In addition, there are now a range of senior clinical posts (for example, advanced practitioners and nurse consultants) for which Master's level qualifications are required. Most Master's degree courses are part time and are classified as taught courses, as for example the MA or MSc, or are obtained by research, that is MPhil. Distance learning is also an available mode of study (currently through the Institute of Nursing, RCN London – see Appendix).

Table 8.9 ENB careers networking facility – post-registration opportunities

- Community nursing
- Framework and Higher Award
- Practice nursing
- Health visiting
- School nursing
- Occupational health nursing
- Midwifery
- Diploma in Nursing Studies
- Community psychiatric nursing
- Teacher preparation

It is not enough to focus on professional and academic requirements in isolation from personal work and family needs – these will now be explored in turn.

Personal and work needs and career choices

Schober (1990) identified a range of personal needs relating to professional career development as follows:

- job satisfaction;
- job security;
- status of the role;
- salary;
- reluctance to change roles;
- working hours;
- terms of contract.

Job satisfaction is central to our feelings of well-being at work (Schober, 1988). The quality of supervision, morale, the meaningfulness of the work and opportunity for advancement have been found to be more significant to nurses than have pay and job security (Stechmiller and Yarandi, 1992). In Table 8.10, other factors are listed, factors such as those needing serious consideration when embarking on an application as well as contributing to decisions to change jobs or seek promotion. For many, the satisfaction of personal needs may be central to a sense of stability, thus influencing a decision to remain in a post in the long term.

Table 8.10   Factors influencing job satisfaction in a clinical post

- Factors relating to the client/patient group – for example patient dependency
- The clinical speciality and the care given
- The pace of work, for example patient turnover or day care
- Organisational factors relating to care delivery; the dynamics of the health care team
- Opportunities to develop the nurse–patient relationship
- Support for learning, team support and staff support network
- Style of leadership by managers
- Morale of staff
- Team membership
- Opportunities for teaching, learning, professional development and promotion

Family and social needs

There are a number of vital considerations, particularly if you have family commitments and dependants and need to be available for family members. Schober (1990) identifies the following issues, which play an important part in career decision-making:

- the family need for income;
- child care availability;
- the support of partner, family members and friends;
- the availability and cost of accommodation;
- travelling distance from home.

Everyone has their own agenda of needs in relation to working roles. Being at ease at work is closely related to being at ease at home, particularly with partners, friends and dependants. The support of family and friends is central to this complex relationship, and the family and social needs listed here serve simply to prompt you to consider their influence on your well-being. The pressures, for example, that come from financial commitments and the necessity to ensure safe, reliable and caring child care puts many families under significant pressure, which may only be resolved if one parent adapts his or her career. Many women opt for night work to be available for their families during the day in order to maximise their income from extra duty payments. The consequences may be serious fatigue and lack of contact with a partner in order to sustain a reasonable income.

The interrelationship between professional requirements and personal, social and work needs are complex and unique to each person pursuing a career. The demands tend to increase with the degree of responsibility an individual has for children and other dependants. Taking a mortgage on a property demands a stable income to meet the recurring costs, and most of us would avoid anything which would jeopardise financial security.

Changes in employment

Whether changing from being a student on a course to becoming an employee or changing from one post to the next, there are many considerations to be made, which can be summarised as follows:

What are your reasons for a change? Are they related to:

- the need to change, for example following a course;
- the pursuit of promotion;
- the completion of a contract, for example a short-term contract that is not for renewal;
- the need to embark on a course of study, for example secondment;
- changes within the structure of the organisation;
- maternity leave;
- redundancy;
- retirement.

Whatever the reasons for a change, you need all the information you can acquire to ensure you are confident about your position, employment rights and contractual obligations. This is particularly relevant if you are changing the terms of a contract, for example with secondment or being made redundant.

So, whatever the reasons for the change, you need to feel confident about what you are doing and may need support and advice from one or more of the following:

Career advisors	Use local and national sources to check the accuracy of information and the rationales for your decisions.
Line managers	Who should advise you formally and informally about your potential local career and professional development, and give general advice about specialist aspects of work.
Educationalists	Senior and principal lecturers give valuable advice about local and national educational and career opportunities (see details about the ENB career network facility, above).
Personnel officers	Give useful local advice about all aspects of employment, including job availability, contractual obligations, maternity leave, conditions of service and retirement arrangements.
Trade union officers	Representation is often essential if redundancy or a termination of contract is being sought as a result of, for example, the disciplinary procedure.

Managing a job change

Applying for a new post is a significant step in anyone's life. Judging when the time is right for a move or when to look for a new post is demanding; so is feeling confident that making a change is the best decision. The RCN (1995) suggests that the following features are those which will enhance and support the individual at work. It gives a clear summary of what to look for in a new post as well as factors which, if absent, may cause you to consider a change (RCN, 1995, p. 5):

- Nursing and nurses are valued
- An investment is made in education and training
- Individuals are provided with tailor-made development programmes
- Innovation and the development of practice is encouraged
- The success of individuals and teams is celebrated
- Team working and supportive relationships are in evidence throughout
- Mistakes are used as an opportunity for learning
- Those with ability are regarded as an asset and not a threat.

You will see that the concerns of employers for employees are manifest here, as is the focus on support, openness and satisfaction at work.

In addition, before you apply for any post, you need to ensure that you have attended to the areas outlined below.

Background information about the post and the organisation

Advertisements reveal important but usually limited information about a post. Study this well. For clinical posts, look at what the advertisement does *not* say; for example, is there information about:

- where the post is based;
- the grade;
- the length of contract;
- who to contact for specific information;
- qualifications and requirements relating to previous experience;
- hours of duty;
- the general approaches to care and the client group;
- the closing date for applications?

For more senior posts:

- whom to contact for further information and an informal visit.

Role specification

All posts should have a role specification or job description. This should clearly state the purpose, requirements and responsibilities of the post.

You also need to be clear about:

- the grade of the post, opportunities for promotion and how that is managed;
- the system for staff supporting preceptorship;
- the appraisal system;
- the approaches to care and how care is managed (for clinical posts);
- teaching and learning opportunities.

Your referees

You will need at least two referees for most posts. Choose them carefully. They are your backers and often your mentors, and your relationship with them is vital for ongoing support, which you may need for many years to come. They are usually colleagues with whom you have worked and who know you well. They must confirm their support for your applications, so seek their permission and support before you commit their names to an application form. This is a relationship to nurture and respect – a reference is vital to the application process.

For more junior posts, for example, those following registration, an educational reference is requested from the course or programme leader. All referees are asked for information about standards of performance, relationships with others, professionalism, attendance, sickness and absence record and potential for the post.

Don't forget to let your referees know the outcome of an application!

The application form

Completing an application form to a high standard of presentation and accuracy is vital; aim to have it typed unless you are instructed otherwise. A handwritten covering letter may accompany the application. You may be able to submit a curriculum vitae (Table 8.11) and/or your portfolio with the application. It is useful to keep a copy for your own reference. One of the most taxing parts of completing an application form is the section requesting you to explain why you are applying for the post. This is often an open page for you to complete. This is your opportunity to convey to the panel the qualities, experiences and insights you are bringing to the post. Study the role specification carefully and relate your points to each main section, for example clinical, educational, managerial and professional. Include reference to your experience, qualities relevant to the post, special interests and commitments you possess in relation to this field and what you can offer. Draw on experiences from previous posts or experiences, explain deliberate activities you have undertaken to strive towards this position and describe initiatives you have taken relevant to this post.

It is helpful for a referee or mentor to go through this part of the form with you to help you express it appropriately. Many questions at interview stem from this section.

Table 8.11 Curriculum vitae information

A curriculum vitae may contain the following information – it may need to be adapted in relation to the post being applied for

Name
Address
General education
Professional qualifications
Professional education
Present appointments
Previous appointments
Research
Publications
Professional interests/membership of professional organisations
Referees
(if one or more headings are not applicable, simply omit)

Informal visits

Aim to arrange an informal visit especially if the post, location and organisation are unfamiliar to you. For senior posts, informal visits are vital for you to begin to assess the culture, values, staff relationships and resources associated with the post.

Understanding as much as possible about what the post entails and who you will be working with is a positive contributory factor to a sense of well-being about the post.

The interview process

Interviews will be shaped by the seniority of the post and the role specifications. The more senior the post, the greater range of techniques that are employed. It is common, for example, for candidates to be asked to undertake a short presentation of a topic given to them to prepare prior to the interview day. This allows interviewers to assess the professionalism, communication skills, knowledge base and key experiences relevant to the post.

The panel interview

For clinical posts, panel members usually range in number from two to four. A ward sister and senior nurse manager for the unit may be accompanied by a member of the personnel department and an external member from another Trust. If the post involves other organisations, for example the local university department of nursing, senior lecturing staff may be present. Panel members will select a chair and decide on the area of questioning. A range of open and leading questions will be asked, which usually relate to:

Previous experience/posts:
- reasons for the application;
- previous experiences – clinical, educational, management and research;
- features described on the application form, curriculum vitae or portfolio;
- aspects of previous job satisfaction;

- aspects of previous academic and/or professional education;
- the person/role specifications.

For clinical posts:
- what skills you bring to the post;
- what you hope to learn;
- what you need to learn;
- your knowledge of current research relevant to the post;
- what you would do if... : clinical issues/incidents to check and assess your potential actions;
- ideas/opinions about current clinical issues.

Professional issues
- nursing values, commitment and insight into nursing-related issues;
- how you keep up to date and professional awareness;
- working as a member of a team;
- leadership potential;
- teaching needs and experience;   particularly for E
- management needs and experience;   grade and above
- research interests;
- plans for future development/study.

Your open questions

Have questions prepared, for example, in relation to preceptor-ship, orientation to the post, the contract and clinical develop-ments in the unit. This is your opportunity to ask questions to clarify your position, especially in relation to contractual require-ments and responsibilities.

The more senior the post, the more complex the selection process will be. The selection activities may extend over a number of days and, as well as a panel interview, include:

- the presentation of a topic, to an 'audience' of employees and panel members, which is relevant to the role specification. The topic is given in advance; detailed preparation to allow for the time limit given is vital and should include visual material, for example handouts and slides;

- psychometric tests, IQ tests, problem-solving and team-building activities;
- social activities to facilitate social discourse with a range of staff and panel members in a less formal environment.

Post-interview

Whatever the outcome of the selection process, decisions are reached that usually identify a candidate most suited to the requirements of a post. Some decisions are reached quickly, and candidates are asked to return to the panel for a decision. More commonly, candidates are contacted by telephone within 24 hours. Most offers are subject to health and police screening and UKCC PIN number checks.

Opportunities for feedback are often limited, but it is usual for one of the panel members to be available to discuss outcomes and performance, which gives candidates vital insight into their performances.

Not all applications are successful, and there are often disappointments when such rejection is experienced. Reasons for being unsuccessful are often positive and contribute to the experiences of job applications. This is all the more reason to seek feedback.

Accepting a post

Formal offers of posts are given in writing and must be accepted in writing. There are occasions when, despite an offer, a candidate has to decline a post. This creates a great deal of administrative work for any organisation and stress for the candidate. Details must be given in writing and as soon as possible following the interview. Employers recognise that this situation arises in a minority of cases, and candidates must make every effort to avoid this situation unless there are exceptional circumstances, for example associated with health or family commitments. It is recognised that some candidates discover that the post is not what they understood it to be on the day of interview. This illustrates the need to be thorough in the preparation for a post and in arranging an informal visit.

Conclusion

This chapter has addressed a range of issues central to your professional and career development. For the process to succeed, there is an obligation for all of us to attend to the wide range of personal, professional, social and work-related needs that together shape personal development in relation to a professional life. It is not possible to achieve this in isolation from peers, colleagues, mentors, family and friends – on the contrary, there is evidence that this network facilitates the process. Aim to use it wisely and you could reap the benefits and satisfaction of positive personal and professional development.

References

English National Board (1991a) *A Framework for Continuing Professional Education and the Higher Award for Nurses, Midwives and Health Visitors.* London: ENB.

English National Board (1991b) *The Professional Portfolio.* London: ENB.

Manley, K. (1997) 'A conceptual framework for advanced practice: an action research project.' *Journal of Clinical Nursing* **6**: 179–90.

Nurses, Midwives and Health Visitors Act 1979. London: HMSO.

Nurses, Midwives and Health Visitors Act 1992. London: HMSO.

Royal College of Nursing (1995) *A Guide to Planning your Career.* London: RCN.

Royal College of Nursing (1996) *Nursing Workforce.* RCN Factsheet. London: RCN.

Schober, J.E. (1990) 'Your career – making the choices' in Tschudin, V. with Schober, J.E. *Managing Yourself.* London: Macmillan.

Schober, J.E. (1988) The Career Guidance Experiences of Registered Nurses (Cardiff University). Unpublished MN thesis available in the Steinberg collection, The Library, Royal College of Nursing, London.

Seccombe, I. and Ball, J. (1992) *Motivation, Morale and Mobility. A Profile of Qualified Nurses in the 1990s.* Brighton: Institute of Manpower Studies.

Seccombe, I., Ball, J. and Patch, A. (1993) *The Price of Commitment: Nurses Pay, Careers and Prospects, 1993.* Brighton: Institute of Manpower Studies.

Stechmiller, J. and Yarandi, H. (1992) 'Job satisfaction among critical care nurses.' *American Journal of Critical Care* **1**(3): 37–44.

UKCC (1992a) *The Scope of Professional Practice.* London: UKCC.

UKCC (1992b) *The Code of Professional Conduct for the Nurse, Midwife and Health Visitor*, 3rd edn. London: UKCC.

UKCC (1994) *The Future of Professional Practice – The Council's Standards for Education and Practice Following Registration*. London: UKCC.

UKCC (1996a) *Guidelines for Professional Practice*. London: UKCC.

UKCC (1996b) *Register No. 17*. London: UKCC.

UKCC (1997) *PREP and You*. London: UKCC.

Further reading

Department of Health (1996) *Nursing: The Leading Edge of Health Care. A Focus on Developing Nursing Leadership*. London: RCN/Nursing Standard.

ENB (1994) *Post Registration Courses – Opportunities for Continuing Education*. London: ENB.

Hull, C. and Redfern, L. (1996) *Profiles and Portfolios. A Guide for Nurses and Midwives*. Basingstoke: Macmillan.

RCN (1995) *A Guide to Planning your Career*. RCN Nurses in Leadership Project. RCN: London.

UKCC (1996) *Guidelines for Professional Practice*. London: UKCC.

Appendix

Careers advice and information – useful addresses

Statutory organisations

English National Board for Nursing, Midwifery and Health Visiting
Careers Information Service
Victory House
170 Tottenham Court Road
London W1P 0HA
Tel: 0171–391 6200/6205

National Board of Nursing, Midwifery and Health Visiting for Scotland
Careers Information Service
22 Queen Street
Edinburgh EH2 1JX
Tel: 0131–225 2096

National Board for Nursing, Midwifery and Health Visiting – Northern Ireland
RAC House
79 Chichester Street
Belfast BT1 4JE
Tel: (01232) 238152

United Kingdom Central Council for Nursing, Midwifery and Health Visiting
23 Portland Place
London W1N 3AF
0171–637 7181

Welsh National Board for Nursing, Midwifery and Health Visiting
Floor 13
Pearl Assurance House
Greyfriars Road
Cardiff CF1 3AG
Tel: (01222) 395535

Advisory bodies

Department of Health
Quarry House
Quarry Hill
Leeds, Yorkshire LS2 7UD

Department of Health, Northern Ireland
Dundonald House
Upper Newtownards Road
Belfast BT4 3SB

King's Fund Centre
11–13 Cavendish Square
London W1M 0AN

Nurses Central Clearing House
PO Box 346
Bristol BS99 7FB

Royal College of Nursing of the United Kingdom
20 Cavendish Square
London W1M 0AB

Royal College of Nursing
17 Windsor Avenue
Belfast
Northern Ireland

Royal College of Nursing
Ty Maeth
King George V Drive East
Cardiff CF4 4XZ

Royal College of Nursing
Glenbourne House
42 South Oswald Road
Edinburgh EH9 2HH

Royal College of Midwives
15 Mansfield Street
London W1M 0BE

Scottish Home and Health Department
St Andrew's House
Regent Road
Edinburgh EH1 3DE

Useful organisations for career support

Association of Paediatric Nurses
c/o Central Nursing Office
Hospital for Sick Children
Great Ormond Street
London WC1N 3HN

District Nurses Association
57 Lower Belgrave Street
London SW1 0LR

Health Visitors Association
50 Southwark Street
London SE1 1UN

HM Prison Service Headquarters
Cleland House
Page Street
London SW1P 4LN

Occupational Health Nurses Association
c/o Royal College of Nursing
20 Cavendish Square
London W1M 0AB

QARANC
Liaison Officer
Ministry of Defence
Army
Empress State Building
Lillie Road
London SW6 1TR

QARNNS
Matron in Chief
First Avenue House
High Holborn
London WC1 6HE

RAF
Director of Nursing Services
Ministry of Defence
First Avenue House
High Holborn
London WC1 6HE

Scottish Office Home and Health Department
Prison Service Recruitment (Nursing)
Calton House
5 Redheughs Rigg
Edinburgh EH12 9HW

Open and distance learning providers for nurses, midwives and health visitors

Distance Learning Centre
South Bank University
South Bank Technopark
90 London Road
London SE1 6LN
Tel: 0171–815 8254

Institute of Nursing
Royal College of Nursing
20 Cavendish Square
London W1M 0AB
Tel: 0171–409 7365

National Extension College
18 Brooklands Avenue
Cambridge CV2 2HN
Tel: (01223) 316644

Nursing Standard Open Learning
Viking House
17–19 Peterborough Road
Harrow
Middlesex HA1 2AX
0181–423 1066

Nursing Times Open Learning
Porters South
Crinan Street
London N1 9XW
0171–843 4600

The Open College
Portland Tower
Portland Street
Manchester M1 3LD
0161–245 3300

The Open University
Walton Hall
Milton Keynes MK7 6AA
Tel: (01908) 274066

Index

127